Introduction to Community Nursing Practice

Jane Arnott, Siobhan Atherley, Joanne Kelly and Sarah Pye

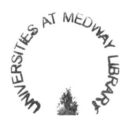

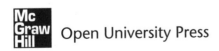
Open University Press

Open University Press
McGraw-Hill Education
McGraw-Hill House
Shoppenhangers Road
Maidenhead
Berkshire
England
SL6 2QL

email: enquiries@openup.co.uk
world wide web: www.openup.co.uk

and Two Penn Plaza, New York, NY 10121-2289, USA

First published 2012

A catalogue record of this book is available from the British Library

ISBN-13: 9780335244713 (pb)
ISBN-10: 0335244718 (pb)
e-ISBN: 9780335244720

Library of Congress Cataloging-in-Publication Data
CIP data has been applied for

Typeset by Aptara Inc., India
Printed in the UK by Bell and Bain Ltd, Glasgow.

Fictitious names of companies, products, people, characters and/or data that may be used herein (in case studies or in examples) are not intended to represent any real individual, company, product or event.

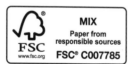

MIX
Paper from
responsible sources
FSC® C007785
FSC
www.fsc.org

The **McGraw·Hill** Companies

Contents

List of Tables

List of Figures

1 An introduction to community nursing practice

L.P. Hartley's novel, *The Go-Between* (1958), opens with the line, 'the past is a foreign country: they do things differently there' and aptly describes the feelings often expressed by individuals when they first experience working in a community setting. Florence Nightingale, in a letter about community nursing some 150 years ago, recognized this difference and identified the need for an added set of skills to work in this setting: 'It is needless to say that a district nurse must be even a better trained nurse than a hospital nurse, because she has so much less help at hand. There must be nothing of the amateur about her. She has not the doctor always at hand' (*Nursing Notes*, October, 1910: 239, cited in Monteiro 1985).

In recent years the community context has changed with a shift away from hospital focused health care to one where individuals experience improved access to care by bringing health and social care closer to the individual's home (Department of Health (DH) 2006a, 2006b, 2007, 2009, 2010). A large proportion of health care journeys begin and end in primary care, with approximately 20 per cent of individuals being looked after by hospital consultants. The remaining 80 per cent are treated within general practice and community services, which is about 300 million treatment episodes being undertaken in these settings each year (DH 2006a). The numbers of individuals working in this setting to support health care has also grown and therefore demands an inter-professional approach to health and social care.

Clearly, all nurses nowadays are educated to a high level and must be fit for purpose wherever they work. However, what still holds true from the above quote is that community nurses often find themselves working alone with families and individuals and must have the skills to manage risk, assess complex needs and initiate and deliver care packages to meet these care needs. In the community, the individual's world comes into sharper focus and the nurse needs to be able to work in partnership with the individual and their family in order to understand and respect the wants and desires of the individual, but also to work through solutions (Arnott 2010).

The aim of this book is to provide you with a text that offers both a theoretical and practical resource as you enter this 'foreign or different world' of community nursing. We have structured the book in such a way so that whether you are a student new to community nursing, or are newly qualified and are starting out on your career in the community, the material can be used as a resource to support your learning and development. We also hope that community nursing mentors will find this a useful teaching resource to support student mentees.

The book is structured around four very different families who live in the imaginary town of Chettlesbridge. Each of the chapters focuses on a different aspect of community nursing and the case scenarios enable the reader to apply new learning to practice, through guided questions, discussion and reflection; each activity is identified by the symbols in Box 1.1.

Box 1.1

Throughout the book you will come across frequent activity boxes. There are three types of boxes with the symbols below designed to help you process the information within the chapters and enhance your learning.

 Reflection

 Question

 Discussion point

The chapters encompass a wide range of topics and provide further suggested reading to build up your knowledge base.

You will find an introduction to Chettlesbridge and the case scenarios at pages 4–7 in this chapter. The case scenarios will be developed further in each chapter as elements of care and professional practice are considered. Each chapter is mapped to the Nursing Midwifery Council Essential Skills Cluster (Nursing Midwifery Council 2010).

The role of community nurses

The aim of this section is to provide you with a brief overview of the different roles of community nurses. These roles will be developed more fully throughout the chapter.

Community nursing covers a range of professionals such as district nurses, community matrons, practice nurses, health visitors, school nurses and community staff nurses who may be found working alongside district nurses, health visitors and school nurses. Each professional works with a defined group within the population: health visitors generally work with children from 0 to 5 years and their families; school nurses with school age children and young people and their families; and district nurses and community matrons with the older person. Practice nurses are probably the only group of community nurses who are regularly exposed to individuals across the lifespan. Community nurses as a collective group undertake a range of activities and roles to deliver community nursing and health care across the lifespan. These activities take place within a range of settings which include schools, children centres, clinics, GP surgeries, schools and the patient's home. Community nurses meet a broad spectrum of needs which encompass health promotion, disease management, community development and public health activities.

The community staff nurse can be found working with any one of the community nursing groups. These nurses usually work within a team led by a health visitor, school nurse, district nurse or community matron, who will oversee the management of the caseload as a whole.

Practice nurses

Practice nurses work in GP surgeries and assess, screen and treat individuals from across the lifespan, from babies to older people. They run clinics for patients with long-term conditions such as asthma, diabetes and heart conditions. They offer health promotion advice on immunizations, contraception, weight loss and smoking cessation and will look after patients requiring wound care or ear care.

Community matrons and district nurses

Community nurses also include the district nurse, community matron, case manager and community staff nurse. The term community matron and case manager may be used interchangeably and in some areas of the country district nurses undertake the community matron role. However, the community matron (often known as a caseload manager) is usually a highly experienced senior nurse and works closely with patients who have more complex health problems (DH 2004). Community matrons work as case managers, providing a single point of care, support and advice for around 40 to 50 patients. They undertake clinical assessments and plan and carry out treatment which may include prescribing, referral to other specialists and services.

District nurses have a specialist community practice qualification and visit people in their homes or residential care homes and undertake patient assessments in order to reduce and shorten hospital admissions. District nurses often lead teams of community staff nurses and support workers. They, like the community matron, work with complex patients and their families giving nursing care, but also offering advice and information as the need arises. The community staff nurse works within the community nursing team, undertaking activities as they are allocated.

Health visitors and school nurses

Health visitors and school nurses are known as specialist community public health nurses (SCPHN). Health visitors work with families with children under the age of 5 years and school nurses work with families and children within the 5 to 19 age group. Health visitors offer support advice to families through the early years from pregnancy to primary school about issues such as growth and development, behavioural issues, breast feeding and weaning, postnatal depression, bereavement and domestic violence. They work closely with speech therapists, social workers and school nurses and play an important role in safeguarding and protecting children from harm. School nurses provide a variety of services such as health and sex education, developmental screening, health interviews and immunization programmes. They too have an important role in safeguarding and protecting children from harm and work closely with other agencies to promote child health and safeguard children. School nurses work within the school setting and often lead on the delivery of personal, social and health education across primary and secondary care education.

Chettlesbridge

Introduction to Chettlesbridge

The following section introduces you to the fictional town of Chettlesbridge and the families who live there. As you read through this section, try to imagine what the different areas of the town might look like and how it might feel living in each of these areas. You will need to refer to this section from time to time as you work your way through the book to reacquaint yourself with information about the town and the families.

Chettlesbridge is a town with a population of people of just over 10 000 people. It has a rich history stretching back to the tenth century and is mentioned in the Domesday Book. The town centre is made up of very old buildings with a famous castle at its centre. The castle is popular with tourists and generates a significant income for the town as it is used as a venue for festivals and concerts throughout the year. Chettlesbridge has grown since the 1950s with three new housing estates. There is a large council estate in Chettlesbridge and the railway station links directly to London and the motorway is three miles away.

The houses within the Castle Close are well maintained under the listed buildings criteria (English Heritage Planning Act 1990).

The houses face the town's attractive fourteenth-century castle, which is surrounded by mature trees, a moat and gardens which are managed by the local council. The castle has a small museum, several administrative offices and a tea and gift shop which is popular with tourists. During the summer months, the castle becomes an important venue for an arts and music festival, and contributes significantly to the local economy. The entire terrace properties are owner occupied; 75 per cent of the residents are aged between 40 and 85, the rest range from 0 to 40. There is little reported crime in Castle Ward; people generally enjoy good health, and the unemployment status of this ward is well below average.

In recent years, there has been an increasing number of new families moving into the Close. Most of the adults work outside Chettlesbridge, either commuting to London for work, or to a large town some eight miles away.

The children either attend full-time care in a local nursery, or go to Castle View Primary School, one of the local primary schools, which is situated just outside the Castle Close. Despite these working patterns, members of these households are active in the community. Chettlesbridge Medical Centre is situated at one end of the Castle Close terrace and provides a range of medical and nursing services as well as podiatry, pharmacy and physiotherapy. The community matron and district nursing team are based here. There are several gift shops within the Close and a small convenience store, which sells locally sourced produce as well as papers and other everyday necessities. The shop is well supported by the immediate neighbourhood.

Chettlesbridge Minster is a large church located next to the castle on the other side of Castle Close. The Minster is a busy venue which not only hosts regular concerts and education events, but runs several voluntary groups which provide community support for older people and individuals with learning disabilities. There is a Neighbourhood Watch Scheme and a Castle Close residents' group.

Case scenario 1

The Browns

Mrs Evie Brown and her daughter Elizabeth live in a terrace of seventeenth-century town houses in the centre of Chettlesbridge. Their home is a grade two listed building (English Heritage 2011) *and is situated within Chettlesbridge's Castle Close. Mrs Brown was a Chettlesbridge Festival Trustee for many years and set up a music prize in honour of her husband who served as a local councillor.*

Mrs Brown moved into the terrace when she married almost 60 years ago. She says she will never leave, unless in 'a box'. Mrs Brown was widowed 15 years ago and her only child, Elizabeth, has recently moved back to the family home to care for her mother, who has become increasingly forgetful. Elizabeth has retired from her job as headteacher at a local secondary school. She, like her mother, is well known in the town. She is a very keen gardener and a member of the Chettlesbridge Gardening Society and part of the minster church community. She is also a voluntary guide at the castle museum. Elizabeth and her mother are both registered as patients at the Castle Close Medical Centre.

Waterfields Estate

To the west of Chettlesbridge is Waterfields, a housing estate which was built in the late 1980s. The majority of houses are either three or four bedroomed semi-detached or detached homes. The majority of residents living on the estate are families with parents who are either working, or retired couples. Many of the residents are employed by local businesses or work as teachers or health professionals in Chettlesbridge or a large town some ten miles away.

The Waterfields Estate backs onto the town's cricket club, park and allotments. The park is a popular area with families, as there is a play park and in the summer there are concerts in the bandstand and the teashop is open. The Allotment Association is thriving and works with the local primary schools and voluntary groups to promote exercise, learning about food and to build up community networks.

Waterfields Primary School was opened seven years ago and is used by the local community for evening events and community meetings. The local Brownies and Cubs groups meet here.

The town council is currently working through plans to build some social housing on the edge of the Waterfields Estate; this has been supported by the local community who have been involved in the planning of this project.

Case scenario 2

Essie and Marvin

Essie and Marvin West have three children and live in a four bedroomed detached house on the Waterfields Estate. Marvin works as a sound engineer for a recording company in London and commutes by train to London from Chettlesbridge. Essie worked as a personal assistant in an insurance company, but gave up her job when her youngest child was born. She has recently been diagnosed with breast cancer and had a mastectomy several weeks ago. Essie has been warned that the cancer is aggressive and the prognosis is not good as the tumour has spread. She is to undergo chemotherapy.

Essie's mother lives in Trinidad and is too ill to travel. Her father died several years ago and her two sisters live in America. Marvin's family live in London but the relationship is strained. He does not get on with his mother.

The children are aware that Essie has cancer but they do not know that the prognosis is poor. The middle child is having nightmares and is becoming very anxious at being separated from her mother. She is 7 years old.

Limestreet Estate

Limestreet Estate is an area of social housing in Chettlesbridge. The flats were built in the early 1950s, originally to house couples rather than families. The flats are situated in a cul de sac and back onto a railway line. The nearest shops are half a mile away and consist of a small convenience store, one fish and chip shop, an off licence, a hairdresser, a betting shop and a laundrette. The convenience store does not sell fresh fruit or vegetables and the prices for other foods, which are mainly processed, are quite high. The nearest supermarket and pharmacy is a bus journey away and the residents collect their benefits from the post office in the centre of Chettlesbridge. The medical practice is two miles away and there is no direct bus route and only 40 per cent of the community have cars.

There is a children's centre which is attached to Limestreet Primary School and the health visiting team are based here, alongside speech and language therapists and children's counsellors. The centre also provides a benefits advisory service and a housing officer comes to the centre once a month.

The local social centre is popular with the local residents. There are a range of activities that go on over the week, which include a slimming club and darts club.

Case scenario 3

Mary, Eileen and the twins

Mary is a 20-year-old single parent who moved into her mother Eileen's two bedroomed flat with her twin boys after leaving a violent relationship. The flat is on the Limestreet Estate, an area of social housing in Chettlesbridge.

Eileen works as a carer and Mary takes in ironing to supplement the family income. The boys are 4 years old and will attend Limestreet Primary School. Peter has asthma and has been hospitalized on several occasions. Peter and his brother Simon attend nursery at the local children's centre. Peter has some developmental delay and is attending speech and language sessions to help with this.

Mary has been on the housing list for three years. She has been advised by the council that there is to be a new housing development on the Waterfields Estate and they are keen to put her name forward for one of the housing trusts properties.

Case scenario 4

Larry and Michael

Larry and Michael are brothers and live in a small council flat. They are in their late 50s and Larry works in a local vegetable depot. The depot owner is a friend of Larry and employs Michael from time to time as a favour.

Michael has learning difficulties and is very dependent on his brother. Larry has a heart condition and needs surgery to prevent his condition deteriorating further. He is worried about his ability to carry on working and his brother's long-term care.

References

Arnott, J. (2010) Liberating new talents: an innovative pre-registration community-focused adult nursing programme. *British Journal of Community Nursing*, 15(11): 561–5.

DH (Department of Health) (2004) *The NHS Improvement Plan*. London: Stationery Office.

DH (2006a) *Modernising Nursing Careers: Setting a Direction*. London: DH.

DH (2006b) *Our Health, Our Care, Our Say: A New Direction for Community Services*. London: DH.

DH (2007) *Our NHS, Our Future: Next Stage Interim Report*. London: DH.

DH (2009) *Transforming Community Services: Enabling New Patterns of Provision*. London: DH.

DH (2010) *Equity and Excellence: Liberating the NHS*. London: HMSO.

English Heritage (2011) Your property. http://www.english-heritage.org.uk/your-property/ (accessed 11 March 2011).

Hartley, L.P. (1958) *The Go-Between*. Suffolk: Penguin Classics.

Monteiro, L. (1985) Public health then and now: Florence Nightingale on public health nursing. *American Journal of Public Health*, 75: 2.

Nursing Midwifery Council (2010) *Essential Skills Cluster and Guidance for their Use*. London: Nursing Midwifery Council.

2   The community landscape

Introduction

The aim of this chapter is for you to develop an understanding of the terms community and social capital and identify how these terms assist community nurses in undertaking their role. You will be asked to consider a range of health indicators that can be used to build up a health profile of the population of Chettlesbridge (an imaginary town in the south of England). This process will enable you to reflect upon the geographical, environmental and social aspects of local health needs in relation to the current public health agenda. You will also develop an understanding of the data which is used to make up a community population profile and how the profile influences the way in which health and social care is planned and delivered.

In this chapter you will undertake a metaphorical bus journey through the town, stopping at strategic points along the way to consider the geographical, environmental and social aspects of the town and how they might influence the health needs of the local population. You will be asked to reflect upon what is being presented to you and examine how these locations might impact on your health and well-being. You will also be introduced to the concept of inequality and its relationship to health outcomes.

You will be presented with a number of case scenarios in this chapter, which will feature throughout the rest of the book. Each case scenario will focus on different aspects of community nursing and help you to apply theory to community nursing practice.

The illustrative census data which is presented throughout the chapter is to help you understand how different factors impact on health outcomes.

Learning outcomes

At the end of this chapter you should be able to:

- define and discuss the term community;
- outline the relationship between social capital, health and well-being;
- describe the process of community population profiling and its relevance to the community nurse;
- explain the relationship between health and the social, environmental, economic factors and health outcomes;
- describe the relationship between inequalities and health experience.

Introducing the community landscape

The principles and theories of community nursing which are discussed in this chapter provide you with the important theoretical foundations of community nursing knowledge.

Community nurses work outside the traditional hospital care setting and find themselves not only working within the home environment, but in range of locations which include schools, clinics, children's centres and GP surgeries. The community landscape is very different from that of the hospital and requires a different approach to nursing. The nurse needs to understand the broader context of the individual's life, and the meaning of community and how this influences the nursing approach.

What is a community?

Community is a difficult term to describe as it encompasses a range of different meanings and perspectives (Arnott 2010). However, community is considered to be of significant value to society, as it contributes positively to its overall well-being and, as Robson (2000) argues, fosters notions of cooperation, cohesion and inclusivity, which are essential components of a civilized society.

The term community denotes homogeneous entities, in which community members are believed to share needs, goals, resources and social and cultural values. Cohen (1985) defines this commonality under three key headings:

- communities of place, where individuals share a geographical location or place of residence;
- communities of interest where mutual characteristics such as ethnic origin or occupation are shared;
- communities of attachment where individuals come together through a mutual agreement, in their religious or political views.

These definitions are not mutually exclusive and often overlap, for example a group of individuals may live in the same geographical area (army barracks), and share similar interests (belong to the same regiment). Community nurses often hold a considerable level of knowledge about the communities within which they work. This intelligence is built up through the everyday activities of community nursing. The routine of home visiting, contacts with schools and subsequent long-term relationships that nurses have with individuals and families, facilitates an awareness of the complex networks which provide support and a sense of identity within different communities.

One of the criticisms of community definitions however, is that they are often developed by non-community members, either for ease of administration, or to assist in service planning and resource allocation. In effect, the defined community may have more meaning for those defining the boundaries than those living

Table 2.1 Definitions of community as defined by health professionals

Definition of community	Example
Geographical	A particular population which is geographically defined
Shared characteristics	Single mothers
Similar interests	Ethnic minorities
An administrative area	A population within a PCT/GP consortia
An at-risk group	Obese teenagers
A GPs list	A practice population

Source: Jewkes and Murcroft (1996)

within these communities. A group of health visitors might define the population living within a group of streets as a single parent community; however the individuals themselves may have little to do with each other; rather spending time with individuals outside of the area. However despite these disadvantages, the definitions as identified in Table 2.1 help to clarify which groups require support in terms of service planning and developing resource allocation. It also helps organizations to measure changes in health behaviours, attitudes and health status.

Questions

- Can you describe the communities to which you belong?
- What sort of communities are they?
- What do you value about them?
- How do they give you a sense of your identity?

Case scenario 1

The Browns

Let us consider Mrs Evie Brown and her daughter Elizabeth and the community they live in. It might be helpful to go back to Chapter 1 to familiarize yourself with Evie and Elizabeth.

Elizabeth has been living with her mother for three months and has made a few changes to the interior of the family house, which have included adding washing and toilet facilities on the ground floor and would like to convert the dining room into a bedroom for her mother, to promote her mother's independence and to reduce the risk of further falls.

Elizabeth and her mother pay for a carer who comes in daily to help Mrs Brown with washing and dressing.

The Browns have always been inundated with offers of support and help from neighbours and friends, and this has enabled Elizabeth to continue to pursue her hobbies and interests.

 Questions

Describe the communities to which the Browns belong.

- How do these communities promote a sense of belonging for the Browns?
- How might these communities help to promote Elizabeth's and Evie's health?

The Browns undoubtedly live in a very desirable part of Chettlesbridge. The environment is attractive and there appears to be a considerable level of resident activity of which they are part, within the Castle Close. Mrs Brown and her daughter Elizabeth are well liked and respected and evidence of this is shown in the offers of support which enable Elizabeth to get out of the house and enjoy her independence.

Social capital

You may have identified that the Browns are part of several communities which include a geographical community within the Castle Close and an attachment community as members of the Minster church. However these definitions are limiting as they don't describe how these networks help to sustain and contribute to the overall well-being of those living in the community. The term social capital describes the pattern and intensity of social networks among people and the shared values that arise from their networks. These networks are built upon shared social norms of trust and reciprocity: a sense of belonging and willingness to engage in civic activity and in turn promote community cooperation and mutual benefit. Putnam (1995) suggests that these factors not only give us our sense of self and individuality but also empower us to manage the strains and stresses of modern day living.

The knowledge of social capital not only highlights the positive aspects of social support but alerts us to the risk factors in assessing needs and helps to identify where duty and responsibilities lie. This knowledge of an individual's support networks is of enormous importance to community nurses as it can significantly affect the outcome of any care package and should be integrated into any needs assessment and care planning. Higher levels of social capital are associated with better health, higher educational attainment, better employment outcomes and lower crime rates:

> life is easier in communities blessed with a substantial stock of social capital . . . networks of civic engagement foster sturdy norms of generalized reciprocity and encourage the emergence of social trust. They facilitate co-ordination and communication . . . Finally; dense networks of interaction probably broaden the participants' sense of self, developing the 'I' into the 'we'.

> (Putnam 1995: 67)

Lin (1999) attributes the link between higher social capital and status in simpler terms and states that the more that is invested in social relationships the greater the return in terms of choice, power and ability to affect change and act as a protective factor against poor health. In contrast poor social capital which arises from poverty or social marginalization has a direct link with reduced health outcome. The key factors which are missing appear to be mutual trust and cooperation within the community (De Silva et al. 2005).

If we examine the Browns' situation closely, it becomes clear that although there is no extended family, Mrs Brown and Elizabeth are well supported by friends and neighbours and are able to make changes to their lifestyle to accommodate Mrs Brown's increasing needs.

Social capital is difficult to measure but formal surveys commonly focus on levels of trust such as whether individuals trust their neighbours, feel safe and whether the neighbourhood is a place where people help each other.

In social capital theory terms, the Browns have a significant level of close net-works or personal relationships and this is described as bonding social capital. Coulthard et al. (2001) describes this as the intense close bonds generally found within families and close neighbourhoods. The intensity of this bonding exists only between individuals in closely linked comparable situations, such as families and closely knit neighbourhoods. Reciprocity is a key component of social capital as it demonstrates the level of trust between individuals and the willingness of communities to cooperate for mutual benefit.

Community nurses and public health

Public health describes the health of the population and can be viewed from an individual to a collective perspective. Public health considers the economic, social, environmental and ecological aspects of health and disease and influences the way services are delivered to improve the population's health.

The following section of this chapter describes some of the key princi-ples of public health which help to inform community nurses in undertaking their role.

Public health is influenced by a wide range of factors which include economic, social, environmental and ecological aspects of health. This means therefore that different sectors of society such as the NHS, local authorities and voluntary and private organizations have a role to play improving public health. The questions below ask you to consider the differences in potential health experience between Castle Ward and Limestreet Ward. As you work through the exercise think about the other organizations that might be responsible for supporting the public health experience within these areas.

 Questions

Have a look at the illustrative census data in Tables 2.2 to 2.6. Try and identify the differences between the Castle Ward and Limestreet Ward. It might be helpful to review the information about Chettlesbridge in Chapter 1 to support you in this exercise.

- How are the different populations made up?
- What might the educational attainment of the different areas tell you about the health and well-being of the population?
- What do you think might be important about the different types of households?
- What might this data tell you about where the Browns live and those living in Limestreet Ward?

Table 2.2 Castle Ward and Chettlesbridge: population (illustrative 2011 census)

Population	Number of people in ward	Percentage of people in Castle Ward	Male	Female	Number of people in Chettlesbridge	Percentage of people in Chettlesbridge
0–4	70	5.8	36 3%	34 2%	579	6
5–11	66	5.6	30 2.5%	36 3%	729	10
12–18	78	6.6	38 3.1%	40 3%	885	9
19–59	500	41.8	260 21%	240 20%	4586	54
60+	480	40.2	250 20%	230 19%	3797	21
Total	**1194**				**10 576**	

Table 2.3 Castle Ward and Chettlesbridge: households population (illustrative 2011 census)

Households	Number of households in Castle Ward	Percentage of households in Castle Ward	Number of households in Limestreet Ward	Percentage of households in Limestreet Ward	Number of households in Chettlesbridge	Percentage of households in Chettlesbridge
Total households	580	8	463	6	7456	100
One person households	75	33	97	21	248	4
Lone parent households	5	14	197	43	998	11
Other households	500	53	165	36	6410	85
Household	**2.20**		**2.7**		**2.44**	

Determinants of health

So far in this chapter we have considered the concepts of community and social capital and how they relate to the role of the community nurse and the individuals with whom the nurse may come into contact. We have also begun to make links between how people live their lives and their health status. In this next section we will look at the factors that determine health and develop this through a closer examination of the population of Chettlesbridge.

Table 2.4 Limestreet Ward and Chettlesbridge: population (illustrative 2011 census)

Population	Number of people in Limestreet Ward	Percentage of people in Limestreet Ward	Male	Female	Number of people in Chettlesbridge	Percentage of people in Chettlesbridge
0–4	225	11	113 6%	112 6%	579	6
5–11	301	15	171 9%	130 6%	729	10
12–18	374	19	174 9%	200 10%	885	9
19–59	703	36	322 16%	381 20%	4586	54
60+	360	18	143 7%	217 11%	3797	21
Total	**1963**		923 47%	1040 53%	**10 576**	

Table 2.5 Limestreet Ward: households population (illustrative 2011 census)

Households	Number of households in Limestreet Ward	Percentage of households in Limestreet Ward	Number of households in Chettlesbridge	Percentage of households in Chettlesbridge
Total households	620		41 450	
One person households	50	8	10 323	25
Lone parent households	269	43	3207	8
Other households	301	49	27 920	67
Average household size	**3.5**		**2.44**	

Defining health

Health is a broad and elusive concept and encompasses a range of models which include a medical, holistic and wellness model.

The medical model concentrates on treating physical disease and health problems, with less focus on mental or social problems and health promotion and disease prevention. The definition of health is limiting as it focuses on absence of disease through the use of morbidity or mortality statistics. The data may illustrate the amount of any given disease within the population but does not describe the lived experience of those with disease (Naidoo and Wills 2009).

Table 2.6 Educational attainment in Limestreet Ward

Education attainment level	Percentage of households in Limestreet Ward	Chettlesbridge	England and Wales
None	24%	0%	29.1%
Level 1	46%	0%	16.6%
Level 2	27%	14%	19.4%
Level 3	3%	17%	8.3%
Level 4/5	0%	68%	19.8%
Other/unknown		1%	6.9%

Note:
Level 1 qualification is equal to at least one GSCE
Level 2 is equivalent to at least five GCSEs at Grade C and above
Level 3 is equivalent to at least two A levels
Level 4/5 means at least a degree or higher qualification

It can also be argued that under this definition, those with disabilities or lifelong conditions are unhealthy; and yet despite this, live fulfilling lives.

A more holistic approach to health might be defined as 'a state of complete physical, mental and social well-being and not merely the absence of disease or infirmity' (World Health Organization 1946: 100). This definition broadens the notion of health and includes the idea of health as being something positive. However, this definition is perceived to be idealistic and vague. Indeed Saracci (1997) argues that terms such as complete physical, mental and social well-being suggest a fixed state over a sustained period of time. However, health is a dynamic process which is determined by factors within and without the control of the individual and health status cannot realistically ever be complete.

The wellness model was born out of a shift away from health being a state, to a dynamic process:

> as a resource for everyday life, not an object of living. It is a positive concept emphasising social and personal resources as well as physical capabilities. The extent to which an individual or (group of individuals) who is able on the one hand to realise aspirations and satisfy needs, and on the other hand to change and cope with the environment.
>
> (World Health Organization 1984: 1)

This definition embraces health in terms of resiliency; that is the ability of individuals, families and communities to cope successfully when confronted with problems and risk (Grotberg 2003), and accommodates the dynamic reality of human experience. However, there is the risk that the wellness definition might be too broad, and what constitutes being healthy is 'fuzzy' and difficult to measure.

What influences health?

As we have already identified in defining health, an individual's health status is determined by some degree to the circumstances and environment in which they live. The word 'determinant' describes a range of factors that contribute a change in health status. The factors which influence health are multiple and include income, social status, education, employment, genetic makeup, lifestyle behaviours and relationships with family and friends and are influential in determining the health status of individuals or populations. These determinants also establish the extent to which an individual holds the physical, social and personal resources to recognize and achieve personal goals, satisfy needs and cope with the environment within which they live (Raphael 2004).

Wilkinson and Marmot (2003) list health determinants under the following headings:

- **Income and social status** Higher income and social status are linked to better health. The greater the gap between the richest and poorest people, the greater the differences in health.

- **Education** Low education levels are linked with poor health, more stress and lower self-confidence.
- **Physical environment** Safe water and clean air, healthy workplaces, safe houses, communities and roads all contribute to good health. People in employment are healthier, particularly those who have more control over their working conditions.
- **Social support networks** Greater support from families, friends and communities is linked to better health. Culture – customs and traditions, and the beliefs of the family and community – all affect health.
- **Genetics** Inheritance plays a part in determining lifespan, healthiness and the likelihood of developing certain illnesses. Personal behaviour and coping skills – balanced eating, keeping active, smoking, drinking, and how we deal with life's stresses and challenges – all affect health.
- **Health services** Access and use of services that prevent and treat disease influence health.
- **Gender** Men and women suffer from different types of diseases at different ages.

If we reflect on the Browns, it is clear that Mrs Brown and her daughter live a comparatively comfortable life, despite Mrs Brown's increasing care needs. Indeed life expectancy at birth is higher in Castle Ward than anywhere else in Chettlesbridge. Male life expectancy is 78 years in Castle Ward compared to 73 years in Limestreet Ward, the poorest ward in Chettlesbridge, and indeed the county. For women the gap is even greater, with females enjoying at least six years more life at 81 years in Castle Ward compared to 75 years in Limestreet Ward. This would indicate that the environment and life that the Browns live is conducive to a healthy life. The Browns have sufficient funds to buy in support and adjust their immediate living environment as necessary. In other words they have a degree of autonomy and choice over how they live their lives.

Let's look at two other families, who live on the Limestreet Estate in Chettlesbridge and consider how their environment and circumstances impact on their health and how much autonomy and choice they have to improve their health. We have already identified that life expectancy is shorter in Limestreet compared to Castle Ward, and that it is ranked as one of the most socially deprived areas in the county.

Case scenario 2

Mary and Eileen

6b Orchard Flats

Mary is a 20-year-old single parent who moved into her mother Eileen's two bedroomed flat with her twin boys after leaving a violent relationship. The flat is on the Limestreet Estate, an area of social housing in Chettlesbridge.

Mary's partner Paul left when the boys were a few months old. He was a heavy drinker and was prone to violent outbursts. Mary disclosed to the health visitor that she was frightened for her own and her children's safety and consented to a referral to social services for support. Paul is currently serving a two year sentence for burglary and Mary is concerned that he may cause trouble when he is released. She has regular contact with the family health visitor and has shared her recent concerns.

Eileen is a heavy smoker and Mary finds this difficult as it aggravates Peter's asthma. Mary feels trapped as she relies on her mother and she doesn't want to upset her, but is worried about Peter's health. Mary also relies heavily on her mother for social support. She does attend some groups at the local children's centre with the twins, but finds it difficult to make friends since the break-up with her partner. She doesn't want everyone to know her business.

Mary has been on the housing list for three years. The boys have nowhere to play nearby. The nearest park is half a mile away at the children's centre. Mary has been advised by the council that there is to be a new housing development on the Waterfields Estate and they are keen to put her name forward for one of the housing trust's properties.

Despite the family's difficulties, Mary and Eileen have some good neighbours, particularly Larry and Michael who live next door.

Case scenario 3

Larry and Michael

7a Orchard Flats

Larry and Michael are brothers who live in the Orchard Flats on the Limestreet Estate. Eileen, Mary and the boys live next door to Michael and Larry. Eileen has known Michael and Larry since school days and they get along well. Larry works as a foreman at a vegetable depot on an industrial estate on the outskirts of Chettlesbridge, about half a mile away. Michael, Larry's brother, has learning difficulties and Type 1 diabetes and relies on Michael to help him with his insulin injections and support in his day to day care. Michael works at the depot on a casual basis and attends a group at Minster church which he enjoys.

Larry has a heart condition which may require surgery. Larry is trying to give up smoking, and has been advised to lose weight and cut down on his alcohol consumption, as he drinks between 20 and 30 units of alcohol a week. Larry walks to work each day and thinks this is more than enough exercise and has been resistant to his GP's suggestion to undertake more exercise.

Larry doesn't like cooking and relies on pre-prepared frozen meals or take-away food from the local fish and chip shop. Larry's boss is always selling off produce cheaply to his employees so Larry and Michael could have access to cheap vegetables and fruit, however Larry doesn't enjoy cooking and when he does allow Michael to cook, Larry gets impatient with the mess and time it takes.

Michael also belongs to a support group and grows vegetables as part of the group's activities. Sometimes he cooks with the group helpers, or gives the vegetables to the neighbours Eileen and Mary. On occasions, Eileen will invite Larry and Michael in for a meal.

The brothers like their flat as it is comfortable and their neighbours are friendly. Larry and Michael and Eileen go to a local club twice a week, as Larry and Eileen are members of the local darts team.

Questions

Go back to the description of Castle Ward and then compare that with the description of Limestreet Ward.

- What differences can you identify between Castle Ward and Limestreet Ward? How might these differences impact on the two different families living in Orchard Flats?
- What inequalities can you identify?

Inequalities

Raphael (2004) clearly identifies that the individual's ability to change their situation varies hugely across the social spectrum. A lack of income, unsuitable housing and poor access to health care services are clear examples of the detrimental factors on the health of individuals and communities. Marmot (2007) reminds us that there are elements that impact on the health of individuals and populations that are beyond the control of the individual and require government intervention to improve health outcomes; this may include policies to improve the environment, such as reducing pollution, improving housing stock or encouraging recycling to reduce landfill use.

The social model of health developed by Dahlgren and Whitehead (1991; see Figure 2.1) demonstrates the complex relationship between individual determinants of age, sex and hereditary factors and the wider determinants of lifestyle factors, socio-economic and environmental factors and how they impact on the health of individuals and communities. These are listed in Table 2.7.

As we have discussed, the health of an individual or community is directly linked to a range of factors which include where they live, their job and educational attainment. The important point here is to recognize the direct link between social inequality and health equality. In other words, the poorer you are in terms of money and educational attainment, and if you live in a poorer area and are unemployed, then the likelihood is that you will experience higher levels of poor health. Marmot (2007) highlights the need for governments to address the conditions of everyday life that lead to health inequalities, and defines these as the 'unfair and avoidable differences in health status'. Furthermore, the greater the

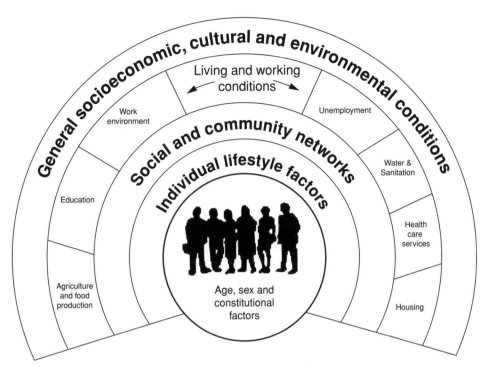

Figure 2.1 Dahlgren and Whitehead's social model of health
Source: Dahlgren and Whitehead (1991)

gap between the richest and poorest people in England, the greater the differences in health status. Indeed, he identifies that individuals living in the poorest parts of England have a reduced life expectancy of up to seven years compared to those living in the richest areas and for individuals living in the richest parts of England, they will enjoy up to 17 years more disability free life (Marmot 2010).

If we reflect upon Mary's case, we can begin to see how the family's social and economic situation and lifestyle impacts on their health status. As has already

Table 2.7 Global ecosystem

Factor	Example
Natural environment	Access to green space, quality of air, pollution
Built environment	Quality of housing, recreational space, safety
Activities	Playing, learning
Local economy	Wealth creation, job opportunities
Community	Quality of social capital
Lifestyles	Exercise, eating and drinking habits

Source: Barton and Grant (2006)

been identified, health and social determinants are complex and significantly impact on the quality of an individual's life. If we compare the differences between the Browns' and Mary's situation in terms of social and economic status there are significant gaps in terms of types of housing, status within the community, employment and power to influence change in their lives. The Browns appear securely embedded within their community. Mary on the other hand, despite her positive relationship with her mother, boys and immediate neighbours is socially excluded from a range of activities and choices because of social and economic circumstances.

Social exclusion

Social exclusion is a term that describes how groups of individuals within any given society are excluded from the networks which support most people in ordinary life (Pearce 2001). These networks include family, friends, community and employment. Social exclusion is a broad concept where individuals are disenfranchised through deprivation, stigma, isolation and failures in social protection. Social exclusion usually falls into three categories: exclusion identified with poverty; exclusion identified with unemployment; and exclusion which comes about through being a part of a stigmatized group. This might include someone with mental ill health, a pregnant teenager and an individual with a physical disability or learning difficulty. If we examine Mary's situation, it is evident that her circumstances impact on her ability to engage in society. Mary is currently unemployed, has few academic qualifications and is caring for two young children in less than ideal circumstances. Mary was considered to be an able student but her relationship with Paul interfered with her schooling.

Mary has attended several courses at the local children's centre. Mary has also considered applying to undertake various courses but the cost in terms of travel and child care are prohibitive. Mary has decided to delay her application until the boys are at school as she wishes to look after them and not rely on extra child care.

Michael is very reliant on his brother for his social support and has neighbours who have known him for many years and will 'keep an eye out' for him. Michael also attends a community support group and helps out at Larry's work. However, without these networks and support systems, Michael is at risk of becoming socially isolated. Larry is solely responsible for Michael's care since their mother died and relies on Eileen, their neighbour, for emotional support.

Housing

Poor housing stock has been attributed to a range of poor health and social outcomes (Graham 2004). Individuals and principally those who are very elderly, young or have some form of chronic illness will be at particular risk. People who live in damp, overcrowded housing are more likely to experience higher levels of stress, mental health problems and physical ill health, including chronic respiratory conditions. Mayor (2004) identifies that the impact for children living in such conditions places them at greater risk of developing specific illnesses; one in 12 children will develop respiratory diseases such as asthma, bronchitis or tuberculosis and there is a significantly increased risk of developing meningitis.

The long-term effects for children living in overcrowded conditions affects their ability to learn which can have a lasting impact on their ability to succeed in later life (Harker 2006). Furthermore, the roots of offending and behavioural difficulties are often associated with the stress of living in poor housing (Friedman 2010).

Poor housing costs the National Health Service £2.5 billion a year and chronic long-term illness such as asthma and bronchitis is associated with poor school attendance and educational attainment (Friedman 2010). The social and physical characteristics of the environment is vital in maintaining good health, however poor quality housing is often situated in impoverished areas, with few local amenities such as medical services, shopping centres and leisure facilities.

Mary's housing situation is problematic. Most people in the Limestreet Estate rent accommodation compared to Castle Ward, where it is mostly owner occupied. There are four people living in a small flat which was built for couples without children. In Castle Ward the average house occupancy is 2.28 people living in a four bedroomed property; compared to 3.5 people sharing three bedroomed rented accommodation. Mary's flat is overcrowded and there is evidence of damp in the bedrooms. Numerous calls and letters from the health visitor, social worker and GP to the local housing department have been made but nothing has been done to resolve this. The flat backs onto a railway line, which links to London. Trains pass through Chettlesbridge four times an hour. There have been concerns about the noise levels and more worryingly children from the estate have been found playing near the line. Mary does her best to get the boys out to play, but the small grassed area outside the flats is unsafe because dog owners regularly allow their dogs to foul here.

The impact of living on the Limestreet Estate for Mary and her family is significant. Peter is often unwell and regularly attends the Castle Medical Centre and on a few occasions has been hospitalized in order to stabilize his asthma. When Peter needs hospitalization, Mary has to make the journey to the District General Hospital some 15 miles away. Mary is very careful with money, but finds the cost of travel eats into her tight budget. Eileen helps her daughter out with transport as much as she can, but has to accept work when it is offered.

Smoking

Smoking rates in Limestreet Ward are significantly higher than anywhere else in Chettlesbridge with a corresponding higher incidence of cardiac heart disease, asthma and chronic obstructive pulmonary disease (COPD). Although there is research linking increased rates of respiratory illness in children to poor housing, there is also a clear correlation between passive smoking and associated diseases, such as asthma and bronchitis (The NHS information Centre for Health and Social Care 2010).

Passive smoking has been shown to have lifelong effects on children's health. Children who grow up with parents or siblings who smoke are 90 per cent more likely to smoke (The NHS Information Centre for Health and Social Care 2010) and for children who go on to be non-smoking adults the ongoing risk to their health from childhood exposure to passive smoking is significant (Ferrence 2010).

Smoking is inextricably linked to social deprivation. Research demonstrates that smoking rates increase across the social spectrum. In 2009, 26 per cent of manual workers smoked in comparison to 16 per cent of those within non-manual households (The NHS Information Centre for Health and Social Care 2010). Smoking is the major risk factor for cardio vascular disease (CVD) in adults, causing approximately 25 000 deaths per year. Furthermore, Action on Smoking (2011) estimates that one in five premature deaths related to CVD is smoking related. Smoking not only significantly impacts on life expectancy, but is strongly associated with increased mortality rates of certain cancers and chronic pulmonary disease. There is also research to indicate that for those who smoke heavily (40 cigarettes a day), life expectancy is reduced by 8.8 years and disability free life is reduced by a further 8.5 years (Streppel et al. 2007).

Eileen and Larry smoke in excess of 30 cigarettes a day. Eileen's smoking not only impacts on her own health but Peter's, her grandson, who has asthma and has had several admissions to hospital with acute bronchitis. Mary has recently suggested that her mother seeks help to give up smoking.

Larry is a heavy smoker too, and now requires an angioplasty because of narrowing of the blood vessels to his heart. He started smoking when he was 12 years of age, which means he has been smoking for 40 years. Both his father and mother died of smoking-related diseases.

Diet

Marmot (2010) identifies that the poorer people are the worse the diet, resulting in a greater incidence of diet-related disease. The Department of Health describes food poverty as a significant risk factor for cardiac heart disease and diabetes and certain cancers. People living on low incomes tend to eat less fruit and vegetables. This is partly attributed to a perception that fresh food is more expensive and less accessible to those living in poorer areas. The Food Access Network (http://www.sustainweb.org/page.php?id=234) has identified that between 1986 and 1996, eight independent stores closed each day in the UK, often in areas where there is no alternative. Individuals then become reliant upon public or private transport to get access to food shops. If Mary has to shop at a supermarket, the cost of using public transport or a taxi is about £6 and this has to be accounted for within her very tight budget.

If we think about Mary's situation, her nearest food shop does not sell fresh fruit and vegetables and cheap food is often highly processed, high in fats and salt. Fresh fruit and vegetables have a shorter shelf life which makes less profit for the shop owner. Mary pays proportionately more for her food as she has less disposable income, compared to the Browns who live in Castle Close. Food expenditure is perceived to be the most flexible of the household budget; unexpected costs or bills will bite into what is available to spend on food.

Michael, Mary's neighbour, spends time each week on a community allotment and gives Mary and Eileen an assortment of vegetables. Eileen enjoys cooking and ensures that her grandsons eat a range of fruit and vegetables. Eileen used to work as a cook at a residential home and makes sure that most food that the family eats is cooked from scratch.

Larry and Michael have access to fresh fruit and vegetables but Larry is reluctant to change his eating habits and this not only impacts on his health but Michael's as well. Larry and Michael tend to eat a diet that is high in fat, sugar and salt and that research demonstrates can be linked to overweight and obesity. This is known as modern malnutrition, and is linked to lower socio-economic groups (National Heart Forum 2004). Peterson et al. (2003) identify that for men, 58 per cent more manual workers die prematurely from CHD than non-manual workers.

Childhood accidents

Almost half of childhood accidents are directly related to the physical conditions inside and around the home environment (Harker 2006). Children living in areas of high social deprivation are at greatest risk of accidents because of poor supervision due to the stress of living in such environments or because the fabric or design of buildings is unsafe. There is also a threefold increase in the likelihood of a child being hit by a car (Grayling et al. 2002) as children will often play out in the street due to lack of a suitable play area. There are significant discrepancies between the degrees of investment in traffic calming interventions in poorer areas compared to richer areas of the country, and subsequently children who play outside on roads in these areas are more at risk of being hit by a car.

Mary is concerned about the lack of safe play space in the vicinity. She has called the police on several occasions as children have been seen playing near the railway line. Network Rail's No Messin' Safety Initiative (http://www.networkrail.co.uk/aspx/981.aspx) identifies that 60 people are killed every year by trespassing onto railway lines and that about 5 per cent will be children as young as 5. The local children's centre and primary school have been working with the local council and community to promote safe play spaces.

Education and employment

Poor neighbourhoods are often characterized by a lack of employment. Indeed if we look at the statistics for Limestreet Estate the percentage of individuals out of work compared to that of Castle Ward is quite startling (see Table 2.8).

Table 2.8 Unemployment percentage rates for Chettlesbridge (illustrative 2011 census)

Unemployment	Limestreet Ward	Castle Ward	Chettlesbridge	England
Male	15	1	3	
Female	10	2	2	
Total	25	3	5	8

Furthermore, most of the 65 per cent of individuals in work in Castle Ward have an average earning of £35 000 per annum, whereas 70 per cent of individuals of working age in Limestreet are either unemployed, rely on casual employment or depend upon a range of benefits to support their low income. The differentiation in earnings is pronounced and gives a clear indication of the enormous gaps in personal income between these two areas and the choices individuals can make about how they live their lives.

 Reflection

Let's reflect upon the differences in the lives of Elizabeth and Mary and Larry and consider how income and educational attainment impacts on their choices.

Income

Elizabeth retired from her post as headteacher several years ago. She had built up a good pension and made a significant profit on the sale of her house when she moved into her mother's house. Elizabeth buys food locally and ensures that she and her mother enjoy a meal out once or twice a month. Elizabeth is able to enjoy a foreign holiday each spring and goes and visits friends throughout the year. Mrs Brown has stayed with family friends when Elizabeth has gone away and more recently friends have come to stay in the Castle Close.

Mary's current family income just about covers their weekly requirements. The money she earns from ironing will pay for the boys' uniforms and a few day treats. Mary buys her food from a low cost supermarket and is given vegetables from a neighbour who has an allotment. Mary has to stick to a rigid weekly menu to keep within her budget. Eileen is a good cook and ensures that the family eats well, despite their tight budget. Both Eileen and Mary worry about the heating bills as fuel prices have increased in recent months and there has been no increase in the family's income.

Larry has worked at the vegetable depot for 30 years. The pay is not good but the job is secure and Larry is able to manage his caring responsibilities as he has a supportive boss. Larry is worried about his health and what will happen to Michael when Larry has to go into hospital. Larry does get some financial support for caring for his brother, and some respite when Michael attends his group and the community allotment. Larry and Michael go to the local club three times a week to play darts. Michael spends at least £15 a night at the club on drink and cigarettes.

Education

Educational attainment provides the gateway to success in future life, and if we consider Elizabeth and Mary we can see the impact of this. Elizabeth left school with good qualifications. She gained a good degree and then qualified as a teacher. Mary on the other hand, although educationally able, became pregnant at 15 and did not return to school after the birth of the twins. Larry did not enjoy school and left at 16 to work with his father at a local factory. He moved to the vegetable depot when the factory closed.

Poor educational attainment and low educational aspiration is associated with poor neighbourhoods (Marmot 2010). Poor educational attainment reduces life options and perpetuates the deprivation cycle. Research by Hirsch (2007) indicates that children from disadvantaged backgrounds do worse by a significant margin compared to any of their peers. Only a quarter of children receiving free school meals gain five good GCSEs, compared to the overall population of England. The impact of poor educational attainment is felt across the lifespan.

Health profiling

So far in this chapter we have considered the concepts of community and social capital and how they relate to individuals and communities. We have been introduced to three families who live in two distinctly different areas of the town of Chettlesbridge, and have considered a range of factors which impact on their health and well-being. In the final section of this chapter you will be introduced to the concepts of the health profile and local health needs assessment, and why these are important for community nurses in undertaking their roles.

A health profile aims to describe a particular community or neighbourhood and assists in identifying the needs of the community. Community nurses are in close regular contact with individuals, families and communities and other health and social care organizations and hold a vast amount of information about the neighbourhoods within which they work. This information supports the process of profiling and is used to identify the needs, strengths and weaknesses of a community and to inform the planning of services and allocation of resources

(Earle et al. 2007). This process also requires community nurses to work closely with colleagues from social care and the voluntary and private sector to enable them to draw up a robust picture of what is available to different groups and identify where potential gaps may exist. Health profiles draw from a range of data which includes quantitative health data submitted by General Practice or Public Health Observatories (see http://www.AHPO.org.uk); individual health assessments undertaken within the home or clinic setting; and perceptions drawn from individuals themselves. Billings (2002) describes the use of this mixture of data as an essential part of drawing up a holistic picture of the health needs of any given community.

Health needs assessment (HNA)

In order to produce a health profile, a needs assessment must be undertaken to establish the level of particular need within a community.

Need is a difficult concept to describe as it is often highly politicized and value laden and is dependent upon the group or individual defining need. Furthermore, the assessment of need is often ill defined as those identifying the needs may have a range of views of what need means. Health needs can range from a medical focus, which describes need in terms of a disease or disability health care related need, to a more preventative approach which encompasses social need. Historically, health needs assessment has been top down or paternalistic in approach. In other words, needs have been defined by the professional expert, rather than the community, or individual, with the risk that sometimes the actual need may be at risk of being ignored. Furthermore, when service users have not been consulted in the health needs assessment process, and have been found to be in need, they have felt stigmatized and are often reluctant to engage services foisted upon them (Carr et al. 2007).

However, despite these difficulties the assessment of need can provide a systematic process which is used to review needs at an individual and population level, in order to identify new health priorities and plan services to meet these needs (Petersen and Alexander 2001).

The assessment of health needs not only helps to identify the amount of disease and disability within a community, but also helps the community nurse in understanding of the patterns of disease and inequalities that exist and the impact these will have on the overall health and well-being of a given population. HNA aims to promote clarity of the need and level of need, the available resources to meet this need, and what needs are to be prioritized when allocating resources.

Need

The concept of need refers to a range of problems which people experience and a requirement for some particular kind of response to this need. One of the key questions for a community nurse when researching need is to identify who has defined this as a need: is it professionally driven or does it come from a group of patients?

In Bradshaw's taxonomy of need needs have been described under the following headings: normative, felt, expressed, comparative (Bradshaw 1972, cited in Green and Tones 2010: 208).

Normative need

Bradshaw (1972) describes the professionally defined need as a normative need, which may have more meaning for the professional rather than the individual. However, as Jack and Holt (2008) argue, there is a further dimension to consider here, as the definition of normative may depend upon which professional expert is identifying the need. A nurse, for example, may consider a patient to be in need of a health promotion intervention to reduce high blood pressure. The doctor however, may consider that medication is more appropriate to the individual's needs, and may not take into account the unwanted side effects of some medication and the potential impact on the individual's overall well-being. For the individual concerned however, there may be a range of other concerns which brought the individual to the doctor or nurse and which have been missed: a difficult family relationship, work or financial issues. The patient may benefit from a referral or advice about who to approach for help. The individual professionals may feel they have met the patient's needs; however the patient may go away feeling misunderstood as their desires, concerns and wants have not been considered.

Felt need

Felt need describes those needs perceived by the individual in relation to what they actually desire. If we reflect on the individual with high blood pressure, they may want to lose weight and need information about how to achieve this. The individual may be unsure about where to get the appropriate advice, or know what is available to help them. Until they express these needs, they will not act upon them.

Expressed need

Expressed needs are directly expressed by the individual, so in the case of the hypertensive individual, they might go to a local pharmacist asking for information about weight loss, or attend a weight loss clinic to reduce their weight and blood pressure. Collectively a group of individuals might demand that a clinic be opened at more user friendly times in order for them to manage care or work responsibilities, in order for them to meet their need.

Comparative need

Comparative needs are defined when one community is compared to another. For example, a person with multiple risk factors for cardiac heart disease may be more in need of antihypertensive treatment than someone with fewer risk factors. If we consider who is most likely to develop chronic heart disease, the research demonstrates that those living in the poorest areas are at highest risk, as they are more likely to smoke, eat a poor diet, and experience a greater level of stress (Marmot 2010). However, despite this, those needing the service most often experience poorer access to health care. If we consider the population of Chettlesbridge for example; those who experience the worst health live on the Limestreet Estate and have to travel some significant distance to access medical health care. Those living in Castle Ward however, experience better health in Chettlesbridge and have easy access to the Castle Close Medical Centre.

 Reflection

Go back to the three case scenarios and reflect upon the needs of each of the families. Make a list and then try to organize these needs under some common headings, such as physical, medical, housing and educational needs.

- Identify what is already in place to meet those needs.
- What could be put in place to meet these needs?
- Which organizations would you need to approach to develop services/ resources to meet some of these needs?

For example: smoking rates are highest in Limestreet. Larry's health is deteriorating and his doctor has advised him to give up smoking. What services might you refer him to? The medical centre is some distance away and attendance rates are poor for smoking cessation. Could you set up a smoking cessation service any nearer? What about the local club in Limestreet for example?

Chapter summary

We have been introduced to three families in this chapter, who live very different lives because of their social and economic backgrounds. We have also begun to consider how these differences influence health outcomes across the lifespan; for example, the effects of smoking not only causes serious respiratory illness in young children but is related to a higher incidence of CHD, cancers and respiratory illness in adults.

We have examined how communities can impact negatively or positively upon health outcomes. When a nurse is undertaking an assessment of an individual's needs, consideration needs to be given about the social support that may come from neighbours or groups within the community. The Browns provide an excellent example of how communities can support each other.

Mary demonstrates a high level of resilience although she does not enjoy living in her community and her housing is poor, she ensures that her children have access to the local resources to improve their health and education. Mary is also able to manage her budget to pay for adequate heating and provide a good diet.

The community health profile is a key tool for any nurse working within a community as it not only alerts the individual to the services available for those in need, but identifies the gaps in service and assists in developing new services or resources to meet the needs of a community and improving the public health agenda.

The overall aim of this chapter has been to introduce you to some of the key concepts that underpin public health. You have also been introduced to several families which clearly demonstrate the complexity and challenge of working in this context for community nurses. One of the key learning points from this chapter is for nurses to understand the broader social and economic context of patients' lives and how this influences their health and decisions about their health.

NMC Essential Skill Cluster (ESC)	ESC number
Care, Compassion and Communication	1, 3, 4, 5, 7
Organizational Aspects of Care	9, 12, 15
Infection Prevention and Control	
Nutrition and Fluid Management	
Medicines Management	

References

Action on Smoking (2011) *Smoking, the Heart and Circulation*. London: ASH.

Arnott, J. (2010) Liberating new talents: an innovative pre-registration community-focused adult nursing programme. *British Journal of Community Nursing*, 15(11): 561–5.

Barton, H. and Grant, M. (2006) A health map for the local human habitat. *The Journal for the Royal Society of Promotion of Health*, 126(6): 252–3.

Billings, J. (2002) Profiling health needs. In: S. Cowley (ed.) *Public Health in Policy and Practice: A Source Book for Health Visitors and Community Nurses*. London: Balliere Tindall.

Bradshaw, J.R. (1972) The concept of social need. *New Society*, 496: 640–3.

Carr, S., Unwin, N. and Pless-Mulloli, T. (2007) *An Introduction to Public Health and Epidemiology*, 2nd edn. Maidenhead: McGraw-Hill.

Cohen, A.P. (1985) *The Symbolic Construction of Community*. London: Routledge.

Coulthard, M., Walker, A. and Morgan, A. (2001) *Assessing People's Perceptions of their Neighbourhood and Community Involvement*, Part 1. London: Health Development Agency.

Dahlgren, G. and Whitehead, M. (1991) *Concepts and Principles for Tackling Social Inequities in Health Levelling Up*, Part 1. Copenhagen: WHO Regional Office for Europe.

De Silva, M., McKenzie, K., Harpham, T. and Huttly, S. (2005) Social capital and mental illness: a systematic review. *Journal of Epidemiology and Community*, 59: 619–27.

Earle, S., Lloyd, C.E., Sidell, M. and Spurr, S. (eds) (2007) *Theory and Research in Promoting Public Health*. London: Sage.

Ferrence, R. (2010) Passive smoking and children. *British Medical Journal*, 340: c1680.

Friedman, D. (2010) *Social Impact of Poor Housing*. London: Ecotec.

Graham, H. (2004) *Understanding Health Inequalities*. Maidenhead: Open University Press.

Grayling, T., Hallam, K., Graham, D., Anderson, R. and Glaister, S. (2002) *Streets Ahead: Safe and Liveable Streets for Children*. Southampton: Institute for Public Policy Research.

Green, J. and Tones, K. (2010) *Health Promotion Planning and Strategies,* 2nd edn. London: Sage.

Grotberg, E. (2003) *Resilience For Today: Gaining Strength from Adversity*. New York: Greenwood Publishing Group.

Harker, L. (2006) *Chance of a Lifetime: The Impact of Bad Housing on Children's Lives*. London: Shelter.

Hirsch, D. (2007) *Experiences of Poverty and Educational Disadvantage*. London: Joseph Rowntree Foundation.

Jack, K. and Holt, M. (2008) Community profiling as part of a health needs assessment. *Nursing Standard*, 22(18): 51–6.

Jewkes, R. and Murcroft, A. (1996) Meanings of community. *Social Science and Medicine*, 43: 555–63.

Lin, N. (1999) Building a network theory of social capital connection. *International Network for Social Network Analysis Journal*, 22(1): 28–51.

Marmot, M. (2007) Social determinants of health inequalities. *Lancet*, 365: 1099–104.

Marmot, M. (2010) *Fair Society, Healthy Lives: The Marmot Review*. London.

Mayor, S. (2004) One in 12 children in Britain are at risk of respiratory diseases due to bad housing. *British Medical Journal*, 328: 914.

Naidoo, J. and Wills, J. (2009) *Foundations for Health Promotion*, 3rd edn. London: Balliere Tindall.

National Heart Forum (2004) *Towards a Generation Free from Coronary Heart Disease: Policy Action for Children's and Young People's Health and Well-being*. London: National Heart Forum.

NHS Information Centre for Health and Social Care (2010) *Statistics on Smoking: England, 2010*. Leeds: The NHS Information Centre for Health and Social Care.

Nursing Midwifery Council (2010) *Essential Skills Clusters and Guidance for their Use*. London: Nursing Midwifery Council.

Pearce, R. (2001) Social exclusion: A concept in need of definition social policy. *Journal of New Zealand*, 16: 17–35.

Petersen, D.J. and Alexander, G.R. (2001) *Needs Assessment in Public Health: A Practical Guide for Students and Professionals*. New York: Kluwer.

Peterson, S., Peto, V. and Rayner, R. (2003). *Congenital Heart Disease Statistics*. Health Promotion Research Group, Department of Public Health, Oxford University, British Heart Foundation.

Putnam, R. (1995) *Bowling Alone: The Collapse and Revival of American Community*. New York: Simon Shuster.

Raphael, D. (2004) *Social Determinants of Health: Canadian Perspectives*. Toronto: CSPIAN.

Robson, T. (2000) *The State and Community Action*. London: Pluto Press.

Saracci, R. (1997) The World Health Organisation needs to reconsider its definition of health. *British Medical Journal*, 314: 1409–10.

Streppel, M., Boshuizen, H., Ocke, M., Kok, F. and Kiromhona, D. (2007) Mortality and life expectancy in relation to long-term cigarette, cigar and pipe smoking: The Zutphen study. *Tob Control*, 16(2): 107–13.

Wilkinson, R. and Marmot, M. (eds) (2003) *Social Determinants of Health: The Solid Facts*, 2nd edn. Copenhagen: WHO.

World Health Organization (1946) Preamble to the Constitution of the World Health Organisation as adopted by the International Health Conference, New York, 19–22 June 1946, signed on 22 July 1946 by the representatives of 61 states. (Official Records of the World Health Organization, no. 2, p. 100.)

World Health Organization (1984) *Health Promotion: A Discussion Document*. Copenhagen: WHO. http://www.who.int/entity/hac/about/definitions /en/._.74 k (accessed 31 July 2011).

3 The practicalities of working as a community nurse

Introduction

This chapter asks you to consider a typical day in the life of a community nurse. While we focus on the nursing care of people in their own homes, there are some issues that have relevance for nursing in other settings in the community as well, such as in clinics, nursing homes, etc. The reader will be invited to begin to consider the skills and knowledge required to practise as a nurse caring for patients in their own home. Practical issues such as transport for work, working safely and planning visits will be explored. A variety of skills will be considered briefly in this chapter and then discussed in more detail in later chapters.

This chapter covers:

- transport for work;
- health and safety in community settings;
- the home: a unique setting for complex health and social care;
- skills for assessment, communication, organizing, planning and managing risk required to care for patients in their own homes.

The chapter includes three short case scenarios about the residents of Chettlesbridge to help you reflect on community nursing and consider your own solutions to the challenges presented.

Learning outcomes

At the end of this chapter you should be able to:

- identify the factors that enable safe working in community settings;
- recognize the specific skills and knowledge required when providing care in the home setting for patients.

The themes raised in this chapter should be read within the context of the Nursing and Midwifery Council (NMC) Code of Conduct for Nurses and Midwives (NMC 2008). Sections 32–4 are particularly relevant when considering the risks associated with working in the community. The code states that:

- You must act without delay if you believe that you, a colleague or anyone else may be putting someone at risk.

- You must inform someone in authority if you experience problems that prevent you working within this code or other nationally agreed standards.
- You must report your concerns in writing if problems in the environment of care are putting people at risk.

Each of these 'must do's' requires nurses to be able to assess, plan and act on areas of risk for both patients and personnel involved in their care.

Local health provider organizations may have their own policies and procedures for dealing with some of the issues raised in this chapter. It is important that you are aware of any such policies and they should be referred to while working through this chapter.

Background

Since the early 2000s there has been a huge increase in the type of health care that is being provided in community settings. Many patients who would once have been admitted to hospital or would have faced long hospital stays have been treated in the community, many in their own homes. The momentum for the increase in community services began in 2001 with the Government publishing its response to the previous National Beds Inquiry (NBI). During the 1990s hospital waiting times had been increasing and there seemed to be a mismatch between the number of hospital beds available and the number required. There were many people in hospital whose care could be provided elsewhere. The NBI consultation sought views as to how to manage this crisis. The consultation considered three possible ways forward:

1. to continue delivering care with few changes;
2. to develop an acute beds focus to the delivery of health care, increasing the size of hospitals;
3. to increase the services available to people 'closer to home'.

The consultation concluded with a near universal support for care closer to home. The resulting development of services would see an increase in the number of people that would be treated in their own homes. Chilton et al. (2004) and Pye and Parsons (2008) provide useful accounts of the background of the development in community services and the influence on community nursing. Patients can now expect to receive acute and long-term care in their own homes. This may involve allowing a multitude of health and social care professionals, with their accompanying equipment, into their home.

As a result of the drive to increase the care provided in the community over 90 per cent of all contact with the NHS occurs outside of hospital (Department of Health 2008). This trend seems set to continue with the publication of more recent Government policy aimed at improving and extending community health care. (You may wish to refer back to Chapter 1 which makes reference to the specific policy documents.) Community nursing is one part of a wide range of services that are available to patients at home. With so much health care provided outside of hospital it comes as no surprise that for nurses working in the community no day is ever the same. A typical day for a community nurse might include providing nursing care to patients in their own homes, in care homes or visiting a clinic. The care provided might range from simple wound care to complex care of patients with multiple long-term conditions or those requiring end of life care.

Factors that can affect the daily work of the community nurse

The wider influences of the patient's economic, social and psychological health can all affect how a visit by a community nurse is conducted and what is and can be achieved.

 Question

What do you think may be some of the specific challenges a community nurse may face within a single working day?
   You may have considered some of the following:

- Visits can end up taking much longer than anticipated.
- Equipment is not always on hand and community nurses should be resourceful and develop an ability to improvise.
- Some patients such as those attending minor injuries same day treatment services may not be known to the nurses treating them, and as such it can take time to gather all the information you need to treat them safely and effectively.
- The diversity of people and the variety of health problems and the unique settings in which care is delivered require community nurses to expect the unexpected.

Community nurses have long required skills in adaptability, creativity and thinking on their feet. The accounts of district nurses working in the 1940s–1960s certainly demonstrate creativity, adaptability and resourcefulness (Pountney 2009; Queens Nursing Institute 2008). One nurse working as a district nurse in the 1960s describes how dressings were sterilized by patients in their own homes: 'Well – we had to find a fair size empty biscuit tin, wash it properly, dry it well, and place a mixture of cotton wool balls, gauze squares and various size cut pieces of gamgee in it, then ask the neighbor to bake the contents in their oven if the patient was unable to do it for herself' (Zena Edmund-Charles (MBE), nee Jospehs; QNI 2008).

Although community nursing in this century perhaps does not require the same kind of resourcefulness as the nurses in the 1960s the unpredictability of community nursing suggests nurses working in community-based settings still need to be prepared for anything.

During this chapter you will be given further information about the town of Chettlesbridge and some of its residents. You will be invited to reflect on the particular health issues of its residents. Further questions will be posed that will enable you to develop your knowledge and skills to practise effectively and safely in the community setting.

Remaining professional

Nursing in the community is provided in a range of settings and includes community hospitals, health centres, nursing and care homes and of course the patient's home. It is essential that you are professional in both your appearance and behaviour.

Uniform

Whenever you wear your uniform, whether or not you are acting in the role of a nurse, the public will recognize you as such. Your identification badge should be clearly visible. Your uniform should be clean and smart; and as in a hospital setting when carrying out nursing tasks, health and safety and infection control policies should be adhered to. Shoes should be chosen carefully; sandals and high heels are not appropriate and could be a hazard working in some homes. Uniform and professional identity will be discussed again in Chapter 5.

Mobile phones

You may be given a mobile phone for work use by your employer. It is important that you remember to use it appropriately. Keep it on silent or switch off when in a patient's home. If you are expecting an urgent call, consider the context of your visit.

 Reflection

Take a moment to consider in what circumstances it may be appropriate to take a mobile phone call during a visit.

If you consider it is appropriate you would need to make sure you ask the patient if they mind you keeping your phone switched on during your visit. If you receive a call take care to excuse yourself and take the call away from the patient so as to ensure confidentiality. It is not appropriate to take personal calls during visits to patients.

Introducing Chettlesbridge

The small town of Chettlesbridge covers an area of approximately 11 square miles. The town spreads across a distance of four miles; the outskirts of town cover a distance of about five miles radiating from the centre and the urban area a further two miles from the centre. Approximately 10 000 people live in the town.

The town centre is a mixture of old and new buildings. The two housing estates are situated a couple of miles out of the centre. There is a fairly large new housing estate to the West with good links to the motorway consisting of mostly three and four bedroomed houses. There is an old social housing estate to the East of the town built in the 1960s consisting mostly of smaller houses and flats. Town centre houses are mainly situated in no parking or residents only parking zones. There are several car parks in the town and the health centre is within walking distance of the seventeenth-century town houses and the large sheltered housing developments also situated in the town. The houses on the social housing estate are built with parking located in central areas and access to houses mainly through a series of alleyways connecting them to the parking areas and other local amenities such as shops. At night these areas are lit but lighting is a little unpredictable as vandalism rates are high on the housing estate.

The rural area is defined by its narrow winding lanes and steep hills. During the winter these areas are often snowbound and access is difficult. Mobile phone signal is variable in the rural areas. The motorway is three miles from the town centre with exit and entry points to the North and South. There are two petrol stations in the town and one on the outskirts just before the motorway.

 Questions

With reference to the town of Chettlesbridge, what specific issues might you need to consider in relation to travelling that might be of importance to community nurses working in this town?

You may have considered the following:

- Parking may be a problem in the town centre.
- Safety of your vehicle may be compromised in some areas of the town.
- Rural areas may be difficult to reach in severe weather.
- Lighting is variable in some parts of the town.

How might you minimize the risks that travelling in and around Chettlesbridge may present?

You may have considered the following strategies to help minimize risks associated with travelling:

- Ensure all valuables/medical equipment is out of sight in your car.
- Make sure your car is serviced regularly and is in good order.

- Make sure you have enough petrol.
- You might consider additional security for your car.
- Keep plenty of spare change for parking.
- You might consider purchasing breakdown cover.
- Keep a torch in the car for travelling around at night.

Transport for work

It is important that your car is in the best of 'health' because you do not want to break down at 2 am in the countryside with no mobile phone signal. When organizing your workload the time it takes and the distances you are travelling to get from patient to patient need to be considered. The town of Chettlesbridge spans 11 square miles, with a rural area some distance from the urban areas. Make sure you have enough petrol and good breakdown cover. There are three petrol stations in the town of Chettlesbridge and so it might be useful to make a note of where petrol stations are and which open 24 hours. It is important to consider the safety of your vehicle. In Chettlesbridge there are some areas where vandalism is high; parking is only available in areas where lighting is unreliable. It would be important working here that valuables were not visible and it might be necessary to consider an alarm for your car.

When using your own car for work purposes ensure that you have the appropriate car insurance that covers business use. The Road Traffic Act 1988 requires that all cars are insured (Office of Public Sector Information www.opsi.gov.uk 2010). You also need to check the following:

- Does your employer's insurance cover your travel on work business?
- Does your own insurance policy cover you while travelling on work business? (It is worthwhile making this clear when applying for insurance as not all insurance policies cover business use as standard.)

Information about the tax payable and expenses claimable for using your own car for business purposes is available from the HM Revenue and Customs website (2010) (www.hmrc.gov.uk).

Getting to your destination

Chettlesbridge has some particular issues in relation to getting to where you need to be, which are common to many community settings. Planning your route in advance will help you reach your destinations in a timely manner.

- Keep a map in the car even if you have satellite navigation; technology does have a habit of failing when we need it most.

- There are some areas of the rural areas of the town where mobile phone signal is variable. It is important to have all the contact numbers you may need to hand.
- Before visiting patients for the first time collect accurate information about how to find the patient's house. If referral information is limited, a call to the patient before visiting to find out how easy it is to find their house might save you some time.
- You should record carefully directions or other relevant information such as a distinguishable feature of the house that may help colleagues when they visit the patient in the future. Not all houses have door numbers!
- Chettlesbridge has some rural areas that are difficult to reach in the snow. It is important to discuss and agree a contingency plan with patients and colleagues and that this is recorded carefully.
- You may have noted that parking is not always available close to the destinations you need to reach and there are some areas of the town that are poorly lit. Keep a torch in the car for visits at night. Vandalism is a problem in Chettlesbridge. This may indicate that there are some areas of the town where safety may be compromised.

 Reflection

Take a moment to consider some of the factors that could be identified as a possible risk to your health and safety at work in Chettlesbridge. Write a list of all the factors and possible strategies you might employ to help keep you safe.

Health and safety in community settings

All employers have a duty under the Health and Safety at Work Act 1974 to ensure employees are working in environments where you are not going to be hurt or injured while at work. This includes lone working. The Management of Health and Safety at Work Regulations 1999 states that employers must assess risk and put in place measures to prevent or minimize risk to employees to ensure the health and safety of workers. Policies and procedures should clearly outline the steps to be taken to manage identified risk. Employees have a responsibility to know how to access and understand the policies and procedures that employers have put in place to keep them safe at work.

Lone working

A lone worker is described by the Health and Safety Executive as 'someone who works by themselves without close or direct supervision' (Health and Safety

Executive (HSE) 2009). With the number of lone workers likely to rise in the next decade to meet the demands of increased community services (DH 2008), safety of community nurses is paramount.

Working in community settings you might be working alone in a patient's own home, visiting patients in remote rural communities or those living in areas of economic and social deprivation. You may be working at weekends in clinics run in the evenings. You may be undertaking visits to patients that are unknown to you, patients for whom we know very little about their domestic situations.

When working in patients' own homes the following are important:

- Ensure you have really comprehensive referral information. It is important that you have as much information as possible about the patient that you are visiting.
- Wherever you are working alone take time to find out where all of the entry and exit routes are located.
- Be sure to include any areas of risk identified during your initial assessment and communicate them to all those who will be visiting.
- Make sure someone always know where you are working and an approximate schedule for the day.
- Always try to give an estimated time that you are due back to the office.

The first visit may pose a particular risk as little may be known about the patient you are visiting. It is particularly important that the assessment you undertake when visiting for the first time includes an assessment of any risks associated with lone working and that these are clearly recorded (Reynolds 2009). The Royal College of Nursing (2007) recognize the increased risk to community nurses during the first visit. A manager quotes: 'I feel that district nurses are extremely vulnerable during their first visit, as they are unaware of any risks that may be involved when visiting that particular client'.

Before the first visit, to minimize risk you may consider the following:

- Make contact with the person who has referred the patient to you; find out a little about their circumstances.
- If there are any issues identified that may pose a risk, or little is known about the patient, consider making the initial visit with a colleague.
- Make sure you are invited into the patient's home; never assume that you can go in to someone's home uninvited.
- Ensure you show your identification. Introducing yourself carefully, particularly on the first visit, ensures you begin the relationship on the right foundations.

So far this chapter has explored some of the issues related to transport and getting to your destination and has introduced some of the risks associated with lone working in the community. Using the following scenario you can now begin to consider the preparation that you might make before visiting a patient in their own home in more detail.

Preparing for the first visit

Jane is a third year student nurse working in a team of community nurses based in the town centre practice of Chettlesbridge. The team consists of the following members:

- *Anne is the team leader, an experienced district nurse of seven years. Anne also has a responsibility for the other two community nursing teams in the surrounding area of Chettlesbridge.*
- *Joanne is a band 6 nurse and mentor to Jane.*
- *Paula is a band 5 newly qualified nurse.*
- *Susan and Tom are both community support workers who also work in the team that operates in the surrounding area of the town.*
- *Jane is a third year student nurse on her last placement with the team. Jane is at the end of her final placement in the community and is developing both her skills and her confidence and becoming more autonomous in her decision making.*

Case scenario 1

The Browns

The wider team includes other health and social care professionals, a care manager, physiotherapist, podiatrist and specialist nurses.

At the 8 am health centre team meeting the day's work is discussed and allocated to team members. This morning there is a new patient to visit: Mrs Evie Brown, aged 88 years. Mrs Brown was referred from the out of hours team during the early hours of the morning following a fall at home. Mrs Brown has undergone x-ray to eliminate fracture. No fractures were detected but Mrs Brown sustained a severe ankle sprain and has a small skin tear to her left ankle that was knocked against the door frame as she fell. The referral information contains basic demographic and biographic detail. It also suggests that Mrs Brown would benefit from a visit at home today to re-dress the wound as her sprained ankle was causing her difficulty in walking. No other referrals have been made and Mrs Brown has been advised that a referral has been made to the district nurses and to contact her GP if there are any further problems. Mrs Brown lives with her daughter Elizabeth who moved back to the family home recently to care for her mother.

The Browns are very private. Mrs Brown is an elderly lady who is fiercely independent and dislikes 'interference'. She has been offered social service support, for example for personal care, but chooses to employ a carer of her own choosing. Her daughter has made alterations to the house since she has moved in as Mrs Brown did not want 'any one snooping around'. The house is a listed building, and is typical of an older property; the rooms are small and the stairs narrow and steep.

It was agreed that Jane would visit Mrs Brown as she has been managing a small caseload during her placement and has been assessed as competent in simple wound care. Mrs Brown's case has been assessed by a registered nurse from the out of hours team and her assessment does not indicate any other problems have been identified.

From the information contained in the referral from the out of hours team there are certain details that will help you in deciding what you will need to take with you to the first visit. You know Mrs Brown is a new patient and as such will need a full assessment of her needs. You also know that she has a skin tear to her leg following a fall.

Questions

With reference to the above, what further information might you need before you visit Mrs Brown?

You may have thought about looking on the GP record for additional information.

- Does Mrs Brown have any relevant past medical history?
- What medication is she taking?
- When did she last visit the Doctor?
- Is Mrs Brown known to any of your colleagues?

What equipment/other tools will you need to take with you when you visit Mrs Brown?

You will need the following:

- assessment and care planning documentation including wound assessment documentation and falls assessment documentation;
- consent to treatment forms;
- wound measuring equipment or camera;
- equipment for disposing of clinical waste;
- a range of dressings.

Reflection

Take a moment to consider how you might feel reaching the door of Mrs Brown for the first time, how you will present yourself confidently and how you might introduce yourself to Mrs Brown for the first time.

You may have considered saying something like this: 'Good morning Mrs Brown. My name is Jane Peters. I am a student nurse calling from the health centre. I believe you are expecting me to call today. May I come in?'

Work related violence

The HSE www.hse.gov.uk (2010) defines work related violence as 'any incident in which a person is abused, threatened or assaulted in circumstances relating to their work'. Staff have reported instances of abuse, violence, harassment and bullying from patients and their relatives to the NHS staff survey annually since 2003; the results shown in Table 3.1 demonstrate that this is a real problem. Although the findings from the surveys do not show a significant reduction in the number

Table 3.1   NHS staff survey issues related to violence, harassment, bullying and abuse

	2009 per cent	2008 per cent	2007 per cent
Experiencing physical violence from patients (or their relatives)	11	12	13
Experiencing physical violence from patients (or their relatives) front line staff	15	16	N/A
Experienced bullying, harassment and abuse from patients (or their relatives)	21	23	26
Experienced bullying, harassment and abuse from patients (or their relatives) front line staff	26	28	32
Received training in the prevention or handling of violence and aggression	50	53	49
Received training in the last 12 months	30	28	26
Reporting of incidents of physical violence and abuse	71	71	66
Bullying, harassment or abuse cases were reported	53	53	49
Number of staff said that their trust would take effective action if staff were physically attacked by patients, relatives or other members of the public	56	56	53

Source: table compiled from data available from the NHS staff survey results Care Quality Commission (2009).

of instances of work related violence, the figures do indicate that staff are being trained, are reporting more and have confidence that their employer will act on acts of violence, harassment, bullying and abuse.

The Royal College of Nursing (2008) has developed a tool that supports individuals and organizations in the assessment and audit of risk of workplace violence. It uses a case study approach that enables employees to work through scenarios and consider potential solutions for safer working.

The home: a unique setting for complex health and social care

Previously in this chapter we have considered the risks that may be associated with lone working and violence in the workplace. This section will consider the issues that may arise in the relationship with patients and their families. Nurses must ensure that professional boundaries are maintained while recognizing that by entering a patient's home, you are also exposed to many aspects of their lives that may influence your relationship.

Case scenario 2

Essie and Marvin

Essie and Marvin have three children and live on the large housing estate in Chettlesbridge which was developed in the 1980s. Essie has recently been diagnosed with an aggressive type of breast cancer and had a mastectomy several weeks ago. Essie and Marvin have been advised that Essie's prognosis is not good and she is undergoing chemotherapy.

Essie's mother lives in Trinidad and is too ill to travel. Her father died several years ago and her two sisters live in America. Marvin's family live in London but the relationship is strained. He does not get on with his mother.

The school has been informed and has been supportive and Marvin has met with the children's teachers and headteacher. Marvin has contacted the school nurse and she has arranged to meet with the family.

Essie and Marvin are a young couple with young children, and are both feeling overwhelmed and frightened about what will happen to Essie when her condition deteriorates. They have many questions and are trying to plan for an uncertain future. The children are a little unsettled as Essie has been in hospital and 'strangers' have been coming in and out of the house. Essie and Marvin are determined that Essie will receive as much care as is possible at home and do not wish her to be admitted to hospital.

 Reflection

Take some time to reflect on how you might feel working with Essie and her family. How might you deal with your own emotions?

How might you manage the situation so that you maintain a professional relationship with the family?

Being a 'guest': maintaining professional relationships

It is important to remember you are a visitor in the patient's home, and as such you are a guest; you are there by invitation. Unlike the hospital setting, you are entering a person's home, and it is important that patients still feel that they are at home. As Lindahl et al. (2010) describe this should mean 'feeling safe and enjoying everyday life with family and friends'. Lindahl et al. (2010) go on to suggest that 'the presence of health professionals and/or medical technology might jeopardise the person's feelings of at-homeness'. It is important therefore to always act with respect to your patient's private space and personal beliefs and to recognize the potential influences that may affect your relationship with your patient and their family. Maintaining a professional relationship is paramount in protecting both you and your patients. There are potential conflicts that community nurses have to bear in mind when developing relationships with patients. There is a fine balance between getting too close and establishing a relationship built on mutual trust and respect. There is a uniqueness about the relationship between community nurses and their patients. The term 'professional friend' has been used to describe this relationship and defines it as one that is not a social relationship but not as detached as a professional relationship (Bach and Grant 2009).

Managing your time

One of the challenges that were highlighted earlier in this chapter was of visits taking longer than expected. Patients or their carers may offer you a cup of tea or coffee during your visit. Bear in mind that this may add time to your day; you may have time to accept but in some cases you may need to keep to a strict schedule and decline the offer. Some older patients may not have many visitors; you may be one of the only people they see and they may be reluctant for you to leave. It is important that you consider how you will manage these potential interruptions to your schedule. Being able to spend time talking to the patient is important. This is an opportunity to review their care, providing protected time for the patient to discuss any issues of concern and helping to build good relationships. It is important to ensure that you have time and that spending time with one patient does not impact on the time you have to complete your daily work. You must balance the benefits of staying a little longer with one patient and the risk to the patients that may not get their visit on time. Occasionally a new problem may arise during a visit that you were not expecting, for instance a patient who has been relatively stable and now has an exacerbation of their long-term condition. You will need to assess whether the problem needs to be dealt with immediately or whether it could wait until your next visit. Assessment will be dealt with in detail in Chapter 7.

Patients may also sometimes wish to give you gifts. It is probable that your employer will have a policy about the receipt of gifts that will protect both you and your patient. The NMC (2008) states clearly that: 'You must refuse any gifts, favours or hospitality that might be interpreted as an attempt to gain preferential treatment'. This issue will be considered in more depth in Chapter 4.

 Question

What strategies might you employ to develop an appropriate relationship with patients?
   You may have considered the following strategies:

- Make your role clear to the patient at the first assessment.
- Always work within an ethical, moral and professional framework.
- Be polite, quiet, mindful and respectful of privacy.

How will you ensure you manage time so that all patients' needs are met?
   Managing time is sometimes difficult; you may have thought about some of the following to help you keep to time:

- Plan your time well: estimate how long each visit may take and perhaps identify time for unexpected problems that may arise.

- Keep an up to date list of the services that may help to support to people who live alone.
- Have confidence in your assessment skills – not everything has to be dealt with on one visit.

Dealing with difficult situations

Most patients are pleased to have the opportunity to receive nursing care at home and accept that health professionals are entering their homes. However this is not always the case. There may be occasions where there is a difference of opinion, or when a patient is unhappy with their treatment. Tensions between household and other family members may arise. It is important that you are able to recognize when conflict may arise, are aware of your own response to conflict and have some understanding of how to manage a potentially difficult situation.

In the 2007 publication *You're Not Alone* (RCN 2007) a nurse quotes:

> Attending a remote farmhouse, rural location recently, I was threatened verbally by a patient's husband, *'that he would be behind the door with a gun if he was ever in a bad mood'* . . . this experience has greatly affected my feelings for my career as a district nurse.

Difficulties may arise for many reasons such as:

- patients or their families feeling invaded;
- a difference of opinion about treatment;
- a misunderstanding;
- emotions arising from anger or grief;
- a lack of trust;
- the perception that someone is being difficult.

It is not always as obvious as the situation described above that the potential for conflict exists. Conflict can arise simply when individuals or groups of people have different expectations. People are all different and deal with conflict in different ways. It is important that you are able to recognize the potential for conflict and how you may respond. People respond differently to potential conflict. In the 1970s Thomas and Kilmann identified five main styles of dealing with conflict. They devised a tool, the Thomas-Kilmann Conflict Mode Instrument (TKI), designed as a self assessment of conflict resolution style.

Reflection

Take some time to reflect on the way you manage conflict. Then consider the style descriptors by Thomas and Kilmann below. Consider your own instinctive approach, and how you might adapt your approach to meet different situations.

The five styles of dealing with conflict identified by Thomas and Kilmann are:

- *Collaborating* This is viewed as an assertive and cooperative approach. All parties set aside their original goals and work together to establish a common goal.
- *Accommodating* This involves placing another's needs and concerns above your own in order to maintain the relationship.
- *Compromising* Each party gives up something it wants. This can sometimes result in each party thinking they have given up more than the other. What is being given up has to be perceived as having equal value.
- *Competing* This is pursuing your wants at the expense of others.
- *Avoidance* Not every conflict requires action. Sometimes withdrawing or postponing is the best solution. It is an unassertive, un-cooperative approach; the cost of dealing with the conflict exceeds the benefits of solving it.

Once you understand the different styles, you can use them to think about the most appropriate approach (or mixture of approaches) for the particular situation you may find yourself in. Ideally you can adopt an approach that meets the situation, resolves the problem, respects others' legitimate interests and smoothes relationships. See Table 3.2 for ideas when each approach can be best adopted.

Case scenario 3

Eileen, Mary, Peter and Simon

Think about Eileen, Mary, Peter and Simon. (You may wish to revisit Chapter 1 of the book to remind yourself about the family.)

Eileen has a history of long-term respiratory disease. While Eileen is a frequent visitor to the practice nurse at the surgery, she is often very unwell and requires visits at home to prevent her being admitted to hospital unnecessarily. Peter has asthma and Eileen smokes around Peter. Mary really worries about this as she knows it is not good for his health. Mary and Eileen frequently argue about this.

Today you are visiting Eileen to take routine blood and arrive during one of the arguments. Mary is very anxious and is asking you to reinforce her point of view and support her in asking Eileen not to smoke around Peter. Eileen is becoming a little verbally aggressive, shouting that it is 'none of your business'.

Table 3.2 Use of the five styles of dealing with conflict

Approach	When to use	When to avoid
Collaborating I win – you win	When issues are complex and require input and information from others When commitment is needed When long-term solutions are needed	When time is critical When others are not interested or lack skills Where there may be different value systems
Accommodating I lose – you win	When issues are unimportant to you When your knowledge is limited When there is long-term give and take When you have no power	When others are perceived as unethical or wrong When you are certain you are correct When issues are complex and require input and information from others
Compromising Both win some – lose some	When goals are clearly incompatible When all parties have equal power When a quick solution is needed	When an imbalance in power is present/perceived When complex problems exist When long-term solutions are needed Where different value systems exist
Competing I win – you lose	When time is critical When issues are trivial When any solution is unpopular When issues are important to you	When working with powerful competent others When long-term solutions and commitment are needed
Avoiding I lose – you lose	When issues are trivial When parties have equal power When a quick solution is needed	When an imbalance in power is present/perceived When complex problems exist When long-term solutions are needed Where different value systems exist

 Question

How might you deal with this situation? What strategies might you adopt to calm the situation down?

Westwood (2010) points out that it is not generally people that are difficult but their behaviour. She suggests some simple approaches to manage difficult behaviour in others:

- Control your response, keep calm.
- Remaining silent can reduce the risk of you responding inappropriately to someone being verbally aggressive.
- Confrontation can be avoided if you explain how you feel about the person's behaviour toward you; the discussion is about your feelings

rather than about their behaviour; being honest does not have to mean being critical.

- Listen to what the other person is saying and give them time to express themselves.
- Always behave toward others in a way that you would like others to behave. You are an important role model.

Managing the patient environment

People's homes are not designed for the purpose of providing nursing care. There is no special equipment, no controls over the environment, the residents or the visitors. Environmental risk assessments should be undertaken to ensure patients' homes do not present a risk to those health and social care workers visiting. Your employer as stated above has a responsibility to keep you safe while at work. This assessment will be discussed in more depth in Chapter 7.

Infection control

Infection control has been high on the health agenda for some years. The National Institute for Health and Clinical Excellence (NICE) produced comprehensive guidance for community services in 2003 in an attempt to reduce the risks and incidence of health care acquired infections. Despite this guidance, Gould (2007) has identified infection control as a potentially increasing problem in the community. Issues have been highlighted particularly in relation to environmental factors (Higginson 2010; Unsworth 2011). Invasive procedures, in particular urethral catheterization, have been identified as a potential threat to infection control in community settings (Jenkinson 2006; Potter 2006). There are a number of issues highlighted as possible causes for the increase in the prevalence of health care acquired infection in community settings:

- increase in invasive procedures in community settings;
- reduced length of hospital stays;
- increase in the number of health care professionals working across hospital and community boundaries;
- role changes requiring unqualified staff to undertake increasingly complex interventions unsupervised;
- increased numbers of catheterized patients in community settings.

NICE (2003) provides practitioners with comprehensive guidance for minimizing the number and effects of health care associated infection in community settings. The standard principles make reference to the unique issues you may face when working with patients in their own homes. You should familiarize yourself with this guidance and that of the specific organization in which you work to ensure the safety of patients in your care. This guidance is due for republication in 2012. For additional information the Health Protection Agency have also issued guidance and provide general information on their website for care homes aimed at supporting the effort to reduce the impact of infection on health.

 Question

Consider the visit to Evie Brown – what actions would you take to ensure the dressing was undertaken to minimize the risk of infection?
  Did you consider the following?

- Consider any specific infection risks, e.g. where was the fall? Could the wound have been contaminated?
- How easy is it to adhere to hand washing guidance, where will you wash your hands? With bar soap? What is available to dry your hands with?
- Do you have the appropriate personal protective equipment?
- Can you identify a 'clean' space to undertake the dressing?

Confidentiality

It is important to consider how you maintain confidentiality in community settings. Patients should be able to discuss issues in private should they wish to: often there may be people in the house when you visit. Make sure you ask the patient if it is all right for you to carry out their care and discuss sensitive issues with these persons present. Sometimes people will not move into another room unless asked. The patient may not feel comfortable asking their relative or friend to go out while you attend to them. Discussion with the patient about maintaining their confidentiality and privacy should be part of the initial assessment which will be discussed further in Chapter 7.

Patients' notes are often kept in the home so that they are available when needed. The notes will often contain sensitive information that your patient may not wish others to see. You may have a diary or an electronic device that contains sensitive information about patients. It is your responsibility to ensure that all documentation is kept safe and secure at all times. It may sometimes be necessary for other professionals working with patients to have access to information about them. It is important to discuss this with the patient and gain consent for sharing information.

When considering sharing information with other organizations that are involved in your patients' care you should be aware of the organization's responsibilities. All organizations should be adhering to the Caldicott Report recommendations (DH 1997). The aim of this report was to ensure that where patient-identifiable information is shared between NHS and non-NHS organizations for purposes other than direct care, medical research or other statutory requirement, it is for a justifiable reason. Each NHS organization has a 'Caldicott Guardian' – a senior person who makes sure that patient confidentiality is protected and information sharing is appropriate and in the patient's best interest. More information can be found on the Patient Confidentiality and Access to Health Records web pages of the Department of Health.

 Question

What strategies might you consider in keeping documentation safe and secure?
    The NMC (2008) ask that you keep patient information confidential. You may have thought about some of the following strategies:

- Ensure you have a secure document holder/bag for transporting notes.
- Ensure you do not leave sensitive information in your car on view.
- Keep all electronic devices stored safely out of sight.
- Use a secure password for all electronic devices.
- In the clinic setting do not leave a patient in the consulting/treatment room unattended.
- Keep all documentation of a sensitive nature in a locked drawer or cabinet.

By working through this chapter you have considered the potential issues, have begun to identify strategies and have gained some practical tips that will enable you to work safely in the community. Some of these concepts will be considered further in later chapters.

Chapter summary

This chapter has introduced some key issues for nursing in community settings. Consideration of all the issues that have been raised above will help to ensure that you and the patient are safe and you are able to carry out your role in an effective professional manner, leading to good health outcomes for patients.
    In particular this chapter has covered the following:

- The safety of all patients and professionals working in health care in community setting is paramount.
- Providing health care in community setting presents unique challenges.
- While planning and organization are necessary, community nurses should be prepared to be flexible, adaptable and resourceful.

NMC Essential Skill Cluster (ESC)	ESC number
Care, Compassion and Communication	1, 2, 3, 4, 5, 6, 7, 8
Organizational Aspects of Care	9, 10, 13, 16

References

Bach, S. and Grant, A. (2009) *Communication and Interpersonal Skills for Nurses.* Exeter: Learning Matters.

Care Quality Commission (2009) NHS staff surveys. http://www.cqc.org.uk/usingcareservices/healthcare/nhsstaffsurveys.cfm (accessed 8 June 2010).

Chilton, S., Melling, K., Drew, D. and Clarridge, A. (2004) *Nursing in the Community: An Essential Guide to Practice.* London: Arnold.

DH (Department of Health) (1997) *Report on the Review of Patient-identifiable Information.* London: Department of Health. http://www.dh.gov.uk/en/Publicationsandstatistics/Publications/PublicationsPolicyAndGuidance/DH_4068403 (accessed 24 March 2011).

DH (2008) *Next Stage Review: Our Vision for Primary and Community Care.* London: Department of Health.

Gould, D. (2007) The challenge of healthcare-associated infections outside hospital. *British Journal of Community Nursing,* (12)5: 212–15.

Higginson, R. (2010) Infection control and intravenous therapy in patients in the community. *British Journal of Community Nursing,* 15(7): 318–24.

HM Revenue and Customs (2010) EIM31205 – Employees using own vehicles for work: overview. http://www.hmrc.gov.uk/manuals/eimanual/eim31205.htm (accessed 16 June 2010).

HSE (Health and Safety Executive) (2009) *Working Alone: Health and Safety Guidance on the Risks of Lone Working.* http://www.hse.gov.uk/pubns/indg73.pdf (accessed 16 June 2010).

HSE (2010) *Work-related Violence.* http://www.hse.gov.uk/violence/index.htm (accessed 16 June 2010).

Jenkinson, H. (2006) Is infection in the community a real threat? The example of CAUTI. *British Journal of Community Nursing,* 11(2): 50–4.

Lindahl, B., Lide, N. and Lindblad, B.M. (2010) A meta-analysis describing the relationships between patients, informal caregivers and health professionals in home-care settings. *Journal of Clinical Nursing,* 20(3–4): 454–63.

NICE (National Institute for Health and Clinical Excellence) (2003) Clinical guideline for the prevention and control of healthcare associated infection in primary and community care. http://guidance.nice.org.uk/CG2 (accessed 23 March 2011).

NMC (Nursing and Midwifery Council) (2008) *The Code Standards of Conduct, Performance and Ethics for Nurses and Midwives.* London: Nursing and Midwifery Council. http://www.nmc-uk.org/Documents/Standards/nmcTheCodeStandardsofConductPerformanceAndEthicsForNursesAndMidwives_LargePrintVersion.PDF (accessed 16 June 2010).

Office of Public Sector Information (2010) Road Traffic Act 1988. http://www.opsi.gov.uk/acts/acts1988/ukpga_19880052_en_1 (accessed 16 June 2010).

Potter, J. (2006) Risks of long-term catheterization in the community – and managing them. *British Journal of Community Nursing,* 11(9): 370–3.

Pountney, D. (2009) Then and now: a day in the life of the district nurse. *British Journal of Community Nursing*, 14(4): 162–4.

Pye, S. and Parsons, J. (2008) The development of outpatient and day services in primary care. In: L. Howartson-Jones and P. Ellis (eds) *Outpatient, Day Surgery and Ambulatory Care*. Oxford: Wiley-Blackwell.

QNI (Queens Nursing Institute) (2008) http://www.districtnursing150.org.uk/ (accessed 8 June 2010).

RCN (Royal College of Nursing) (2007) *You're Not Alone. The RCN – Campaigning to Protect Lone Workers*. London: Royal College of Nursing.

RCN (2008) *Work Related Violence: An RCN Tool to Manage Risk and Promote Safer Working Practices in Healthcare*. http://www.rcn.org.uk/_data/assets/pdf_file/ 0010/192493/003271.pdf (accessed 12 March 2011).

Reynolds, J. (2009) Undertaking risk management in community nursing practice. *Journal of Community Nursing*, 23(11): 24–8.

Unsworth, J. (2011) District nurses' and aseptic technique: where did it all go wrong? *British Journal of Community Nursing*, 16(1): 30–4.

Westwood, C. (2010) Managing difficult behaviour. *Nursing Management – UK*, 17(6): 20–1.

Further reading

Bach, S. and Grant, A. (2009) *Communication and Interpersonal Skills for Nurses*. Exeter: Learning Matters.

Griffith, R. and Tengnah, C. (2010) *Law and Professional Issues in Nursing*. Exeter: Learning Matters.

Useful websites

Department of Health http://www.dh.gov.uk
Health and Safety Executive http://www.hse.gov.uk/index.htm
Health Protection Agency http://www.hpa.org.uk
Mind Tools http://www.mindtools.com
NHS Business Services Authority http://www.nhsbsa.nhs.uk/Index.aspx
Nursing and Midwifery Council http://www.nmc-uk.org
Royal College of Nursing http://www.rcn.org.uk/

4 Working with vulnerable groups

Introduction

This chapter will provide an overview of the terms 'vulnerable adult or child' and what this means in present day society and the serious impact this status can have upon an individual's health and well-being. Nurses and other health and social care professionals have a key role in the care of adults and children who would be considered vulnerable. The Nursing and Midwifery Council *The Code: Standards of Conduct, Performance And Ethics For Nurses And Midwives* (2008) sets down some key principles in protecting individuals from risk and harm, and therefore in order to fulfil this role, it is important that you not only understand what is meant by the term 'vulnerable adult or child', but know how to recognize when an individual is at risk or being harmed, abused or neglected and what to do.

We will focus on three of the case scenarios within this chapter: Larry and Michael, the Browns, and Mary and her twins. We will explore the factors that may indicate that these individuals are potentially vulnerable. You will be asked to consider the risk factors and explore possible solutions through a series of reflective exercises. The reflective process will enable you to identify the roles and responsibilities of different professionals, agencies and families concerned with protecting an individual from harm. It is envisaged that this approach will allow you to reflect upon your feelings and views about this area of practice.

Although there are some similarities in the definitions of the vulnerable adult and child, there are also distinctive differences in the way adult and child vulnerability is defined and managed and therefore the chapter will divide into two parts. Part One will consider the vulnerable adult and Part Two will examine issues relating to vulnerable children. The final part of the chapter draws the themes discussed together, identifying the key issues for social and health care professionals working with these issues.

Learning outcomes

At the end of this chapter you should be able to:

- define the terms vulnerable adult and vulnerable child and identify the underlying contributory factors which may lead to vulnerability;
- describe the term abuse and the different types of abuse an adult or child may experience. Consider how this is managed as part of an assessment;

- examine some of the key legislation which protects vulnerable individuals and describe how this relates to the role and responsibilities of the nurse and other health and social care professionals;
- identify the protocols for referral to other agencies.

Part one: vulnerable adults

Safeguarding activities are key in preventing harm to individuals and populations. These activities are wide ranging and nurses need to be aware of them in order to understand their role in promoting patients' welfare. However, individuals become vulnerable and at risk of harm for other reasons and the next section discusses what it means to be a vulnerable adult and what is in place to support and protect such individuals from risk of harm.

What is a vulnerable adult?

Brown (2010) discusses the use of many terms that have been used to describe what we now term a vulnerable adult since the 1970s. Brown (2010) goes on to discuss how the protection of adults has developed, with the publication of the 1993 Action on Elder Abuse (www.elderabuse.org.uk) and subsequent adoption of the term elder abuse by the World Health Organization (WHO) (www.who.int 2011). WHO defines the abuse of older people – 'elder abuse' – as: 'a single, or repeated act, or lack of appropriate action, occurring within any relationship where there is an expectation of trust which causes harm or distress to an older person'.

This definition has been broadened to encompass other vulnerable adult groups and has been further described in *No Secrets* (DH 2000) and defines a vulnerable adult as:

> a person aged 18 or over who is or maybe in need of community care services (all care services provided in any setting or context) by reason of mental or other disability, age or illness and who is or maybe unable to take care of him or herself, or unable to protect him or herself against significant harm or serious exploitation.

Let's consider how the *No Secrets* (DH 2000) definition might relate to Michael and Larry's situation.

Michael is very friendly and while the local residents know him well and take care of him, he has occasionally boarded the local bus and has been found in the adjoining villages to Chettlesbridge, unaware of potential danger.

Michael is very trusting and enjoys being out and about in the town. He is often found in conversation with visitors to the town who he does not know. Most people treat Michael well, but he has been verbally abused on one or two occasions by a local gang on the Limestreet Estate and the local community support officer has been involved.

Michael has Type 1 diabetes and is dependent on Larry to help him with his insulin injections and to manage his diet. Michael can get aggressive when his blood sugar levels

*are not well controlled and this has occurred on several occasions recently when Michael
has refused to eat. He says he is frightened and doesn't want Larry to go into hospital.*

*Larry is due to have surgery and Michael's social worker is due to visit the brothers to
assess how best to support Michael through this period. Michael and Larry have had lots
of offers from their friends to help out.*

Reflection

Read through the case scenario again and identify any potential risks to the
individuals within the case scenario.

- List the concerns under a range of categories.
- Who might you approach to discuss these concerns?
- What are Michael and Larry's roles in this?

Write up some notes as we will come back to this exercise later in the chapter
and will review some possible solutions.

The policy background

In 1998 the Government recognized that previous systems to safeguard vulnerable adults were not strong enough. In its White Paper *Modernising Social Services*
(DH 1998) the Government pledged to improve the protection of people needing
care support. In 2000 the publication of *No Secrets* gave guidance to all statutory
agencies for the development of 'codes of practice' that would provide protection
for vulnerable adults. The development of policies to protect vulnerable adults
has been led by local authorities social services departments. Since the publication of *No Secrets* (DH 2000) there have been several changes to the way in which
vulnerable groups including adults are protected. In 2005 the publication of a
National Framework Document *Safeguarding Adults* (Association of Social Services
Directors 2005) provided good practice standards for all those agencies involved
in the continuing development of processes designed to protect vulnerable adults.
The framework provided guidance for both the implementation and audit of the
standards.

Further to the publication of *No Secrets* (DH 2000) a review was held in 2008,
the 'Report on the consultation of the review of No Secrets' (DH 2009) identified
that the systems in place for protecting vulnerable adults required improvement
within the NHS. The need to consider the relationship between protection of vulnerable adults, clinical incident reporting, complaints and issues concerning safety
should be considered in the wider context of adult protection. Further guidance
to support NHS organizations to fully integrate policies and procedures for reporting clinical incidents and raising issues about adult protection was published in
Clinical Governance and Adult Safeguarding (DH 2010). The publication intends to

provide clear guidance for reporting and to support improved partnership working across agencies involved in the protection of vulnerable adults. Specific guidance for health services practitioners has been published by the Department of Health (2011). Both these publications provide a framework from which organizations involved in caring for vulnerable adults are able to design robust processes for the identification, management and prevention of harm. There is a useful flow chart that identifies three initial steps to be taken to protect vulnerable adults. These steps are outlined as:

- Event – the identification of a concern;
- Report – letting someone else know about the event by whatever means the organization provides;
- Review – this process aims to decide whether the event should be considered within the safeguarding adults procedures – is this event a safeguarding issue?

Questions

- Are you aware of your organization's safeguarding policies and procedures?
- Who would you approach in your organization if you had concerns?

A study in the south-east of England found that referrals for adult protection had increased between 1998 and 2005 (Mansell et al. 2009). Robust processes were found to be a contributory factor in this study.

Reflection

Let's reflect upon the potential risks you identified for Michael in the Reflection on page 57 and then explore what might be done next by following part one of the three step process above.

Michael: identification of a concern

Main concern

Michael will become significantly more vulnerable if support is not put in place when Larry is in hospital as Michael requires 24-hour supervision and is dependent upon his brother for his day to day care. Support will need to be continued after Larry's discharge as Larry will need several weeks to recuperate.

Identify further concerns:

- **medical issues:** Type 1 diabetic: insulin, blood sugars, diet;
- **social issues:** Mental Health Capacity Act (2005) Lack of social boundaries, unaware of potential risk of strangers; maintenance of regular routine: attend weekly activities;
- **emotional and psychological issues:** increased anxiety about Larry's hospitalization; refusal to eat.

Larry and Michael are well known to the Castle Ward Medical Practice and are visited from time to time by one of the social workers from the Adult Learning Disabilities Team. The social worker has suggested to Larry and Michael that they meet with the community nursing team and one of the practice nurses and GPs from Castle Ward to see how best the brothers can be supported.

One of the key issues for everyone involved in this case is to ensure that Michael is helped to understand what will happen to Larry and how Michael and Larry will be supported through this stressful time. The Mental Health Capacity Act (2005) sets out a structure to support individuals such as Michael in deciding how their care is planned.

Larry and Michael ask Eileen their neighbour to attend the meeting as well, as Michael and Eileen have a very good relationship and she has offered to support Michael when Larry is in hospital.

The meeting takes place and Michael's main concern is that he doesn't know how long Larry will be away from home. The GP and the social worker are able to reassure Michael that Larry will be away for about two days. Michael makes it very clear that he doesn't want to go into care and wants to stay at home. It appears that this is Michael's main fear and worry.

The following plan is put in place:

Eileen will stay with Michael when Larry is in hospital. She will also ensure that Michael attends his usual weekly activities.

The social worker will organize for a member of her team to contact Eileen to offer daily support and if Michael would like to attend his group activities on a daily basis during Larry's recuperation, then this can be arranged. The social worker will organize transport to help Eileen if necessary or fund some of Eileen's petrol costs.

A community nurse will be asked to review Michael's diabetes over the next few weeks; since his eating has become erratic, his blood sugars have been unstable.

The community nursing team will be visiting Larry at home after his operation. The community nurse suggests that the brothers might like to stock up on prepared meals to reduce the stress for Larry and to ensure that Michael has access to nutritious food.

A further meeting is arranged for two weeks after Larry's operation to monitor the situation.

Eileen and Larry are advised about whom to contact should Michael become distressed. They are also given Out of Hours contact details.

By the end of the meeting Michael appears to be calmer. He thanks Eileen for her offer to stay with him.

Questions

- What do you think about this plan?
- Do you think it meets the needs of the brothers?
- What about Eileen, is it right for her to undertake this role?

Protecting vulnerable adults – the law

In 2006 the Safeguarding Vulnerable Groups Act came into force providing additional legal protection for vulnerable adults. The tragic murders of Jessica Chapman and Holly Wells in 2002 prompted the Bichard Inquiry in which the issue of the recruitment of people working with vulnerable groups were not robust enough. The recommendations from the report included the development of a 'vetting and barring' scheme which is currently under review. The scheme formed part of the role of the Independent Safeguarding Authority (ISA) and helped employers in making the decision as to whether it is safe to employ an applicant to a job where vulnerable groups may be at risk.

Questions

Go to the ISA website (http://www.isa.homeoffice.gov.uk/).

- What does an employer need to do to protect patients from harm?
- Do you know what a Criminal Records Bureau (CRB) check entails?
- If you do not have CRB clearance, are you aware of the implications for you as an employee?

Additional legal protection for those receiving care is provided through the Health and Social Care Act 2008 (Regulated Activities) Regulations 2010. Adherence to these regulations is monitored by the Care Quality Commission (CQC). All health and social care providers are registered with the CQC, who regulate and monitor standards of care to ensure quality and safety for all those in receipt of such services.

Regulated activities include among others:

- personal care;
- accommodation for persons who require nursing or personal care;
- treatment of disease, disorder or injury;

- surgical procedures;
- diagnostic and screening procedures;
- nursing care.

The regulations can be used to support the CQC to improve services or prevent a provider from carrying out any of the regulated activities where quality and safety are below expectation and may provide a risk to any person's health or well-being.

The regulations also outline a set of 16 Essential Standards that can be expected by receivers of health or social care, whether in hospital, a care home or in a person's own home. Standard 3 – 'You can expect to be safe' – incorporates the five standards below. These help to ensure vulnerable adults are being protected through the implementation and monitoring of safety and quality of all health and social care providers:

- You will be protected from abuse or the risk of abuse, and staff will respect your human rights.
- You will be cared for in a clean environment where you are protected from infection.
- You will get the medicines you need, when you need them, and in a safe way.
- You will be cared for in a safe and accessible place that will help you as you recover.
- You will not be harmed by unsafe or unsuitable equipment.

(Care Quality Commission 2010)

 Reflection

Take a moment to reflect on the way in which you have observed these standards being implemented and monitored in the care settings you have been working in.

Now consider some of the concerns that have been raised in the media about standards of care.

Have a look at the Patients' Association website and read through some of the recent reports about poor patient care (http://www.patients-association.com/).

Can you identify the weaknesses in the system that resulted in the poor care? How do these issues relate to your professional code of conduct?

Although the CQC have a major role to play in the monitoring of standards to protect vulnerable adults, other organizations may be involved where concerns are raised. For example the Police may be required to investigate if there is concern that a crime may have been committed. Social and Health Services, as commissioners of domiciliary and residential care, may need to consider specific issues related to the contractual arrangements with their chosen providers. All individuals who work in health and social care settings have a responsibility to the people in their care; protection of vulnerable adults is everyone's business.

Multi-agency working is crucial to the protection of vulnerable adults. Information sharing on a person to person basis was found by Pinkney et al. (2008) to strengthen multi-agency working, although there was some confusion about what could legally be shared. Differences in culture between health and social professionals was highlighted as a barrier to working together and social workers noted a lack of knowledge of NHS colleagues. Multi-agency training has been highlighted as beneficial in understanding roles and responsibilities and sharing skills and knowledge (Pinkney et al. 2008, Day et al. 2010).

What is considered harm, abuse or neglect?

Various forms of harm, abuse and neglect have been identified. For the purposes of this chapter we will be considering the following categories of abuse (Action on Elder Abuse 2006; Griffith and Tengnah 2009; Brown 2010):

- **Physical abuse:** Physical abuse can include causing actual physical injury by slapping, hitting or treating someone roughly. In health care this can also include the administration of medicines inappropriately, using inappropriate equipment and using restraint.
- **Sexual abuse:** This category includes any act of a sexual nature that the person has not consented to: rape, sexual assaults and intimate procedures that a person has not or cannot consent willingly to.
- **Financial abuse:** This is a person's financial security being under threat, by theft or fraud. Older people are sometimes put under pressure or coerced by family members to sign over assets, provide financial support, and give early inheritance payments. Power of attorney can be misused and may be a channel for financial abuse.
- **Psychological abuse:** This can include threatening behaviour or using threatening language. People may suffer intimidation and humiliation. Withdrawal of attention, support or visits can be a form of psychological abuse.
- **Discriminatory abuse:** This includes sexist and racist abuse and exploitation due to disability or any other form of harassment.
- **Abuse through neglect or acts of omission:** This can occur as a result of not recognizing or acting on identified health or social care needs. A person may be denied treatment, adequate food and fluids. Important information about a person is withheld, misinterpreted or misrepresented or not acted on appropriately. Neglect can happen as a result of lack of knowledge or skill – a person may not realize they are neglecting to care for someone appropriately.

Having an awareness of the categories of abuse and being able to assess for risk factors is an essential skill for community nurses. A study commissioned by the Department of Health to explore the prevalence of elder abuse in 2007 (O'Keefe et al. 2007) found between 2.6 per cent and 4 per cent of people over 65 years living in their own homes had been subject to a form of abuse. The perpetrators in approximately one third of the cases reported were described as partners (35 per cent), other family members (33 per cent) and neighbours and acquaintances (33 per cent). Abuse of residents in care homes has also been highlighted recently by Rees (2011) in a heartfelt account of the care her mother received in four different care homes. Milne (2011) provides a commentary on the specific issues related to the protection of adults in the care home setting.

Reflection

Take a moment to consider the risk factors for the Browns in the case scenario below.

Elizabeth has recently had a fall and sustained a bad ankle sprain, is now using crutches and cannot undertake her usual caring duties for her mother. Mrs Evie Brown moved into the terrace when she married almost 60 years ago. She says she will never leave, unless in 'a box'. Evie Brown has substantial savings and as such is not entitled to personal care through social services. Elizabeth and her mother are very private and prefer not to use the services of any of the care agencies, although trusted friends and neighbours do help out with shopping and will sit with Evie if Elizabeth needs to go out. Elizabeth and Evie feel that as the agency carer wears a uniform everyone will think that Elizabeth and her mother are not coping. This has led to Elizabeth advertising locally for a private carer who comes in daily to help Mrs Brown with washing and dressing.

One of the key risks to Evie and Elizabeth is that in employing someone independently, they may put themselves at risk, particularly if the individual they employ has no training or understanding of Evie's needs.

Fortunately, one of Elizabeth's friends is a retired GP and in conversation with Elizabeth discovers that they have advertised privately. The friend alerts them to some of the problems and Elizabeth agrees to reconsider her decision and contact the nursing team to ask for their advice.

Question

How might the nursing team help Evie and Elizabeth overcome their concerns about everyone knowing their business?

What are the signs of abuse?

The physical signs of abuse or neglect may be easy to recognize. There may be:

- unexplained bruising
- wounds
- burns
- scratches
- a history of fractures
- untreated injuries
- weight loss
- an unkempt appearance
- illness not responding to treatment
- recoil when approached.

Other forms of abuse may not be so easy to recognize or assess.

 Question

What signs may indicate that a person is at threat of or subject to other forms of abuse as described above?

You may have considered the following:

Financial abuse A person may be reluctant to spend money, have the heating on in the house, pay for care, wouldn't consider moving into a care home/more suitable accommodation, changes in their material well-being;

Sexual abuse Patients may be reluctant for personal care to be undertaken, be tearful, seem withdrawn, recoiling from touch, there may be changes in behaviour;

Psychological abuse People may express feelings of aloneness, be reluctant to express their needs, express feelings of 'not wanting to be a nuisance, being a burden, not wanting to take up your time', be tearful or withdrawn.

Understanding what to look out for and having the knowledge about what to do if you are worried about the safety of a person in your care are essential aspects of a health professional's role and responsibility. The Nursing and Midwifery Council state that nurses should:

> Have the skills to confidently recognise and effectively manage situations where you suspect a person in your care is at risk of harm, abuse or neglect, including poor practice.
>
> (NMC 2010)

Identify several cases that relate to the community setting and discuss with your mentor how this could be prevented, who would need to be involved and what is your responsibility as a community nurse?

Part two: vulnerable children

One of the key features in assessing an individual's vulnerability, as identified earlier in this chapter, is the degree to which an individual is dependent upon another person for their health and well-being, and the level of protection from potential harm. In the case of children and some very vulnerable adults this becomes even more critical as children, and especially young children, are entirely dependent upon those who care for them to provide a safe, secure and loving environment in which they can thrive and grow into healthy adults. Sadly, as history repeatedly demonstrates, this is not the case for some children, as those adults who are relied upon to provide a caring environment fail to provide for their child's needs and, in some cases, become perpetrators of abuse; the case of Victoria Climbie and Baby P are examples of how unchecked child abuse can lead to child deaths (DH 2003; DCSF 2009).

According to the Department of Education (2010), in March 2010, 46 700 children were at risk of child abuse. There were 603 700 referrals to children's social care services in the year ending 31 March 2010, which equates to a rate of 548.2 per 10 000 children aged under 18 years. One of the concerning issues about child abuse is that children who were neglected in their childhood are 2.6 times more likely to neglect their own children and twice as likely to physically abuse their children, than those who were not. Children who were physically abused are five times more likely to do the same to their own children (Kim 2009). The long-term impact of child abuse is a greater likelihood of mental health issues, drug and alcohol abuse and ability to manage intimate relationships (Lazenbatt 2010).

As we saw earlier in this chapter, the terms vulnerable adult and adult abuse have undergone significant development over the years and it is only within the last decade that these principles have been enshrined in legislation. Safeguarding and promoting the well-being of children has a longer history and has been described as:

> the process of protecting children from abuse or neglect, preventing impairment of their health and development, and ensuring they are growing up in circumstances consistent with the provision of safe and effective care that enables children to have optimum life chances and enter adulthood successfully.
>
> (HM Government 2006, cited in Barker 2009: 21)

 Reflection

Safeguarding children has two key components, that of protecting children from harm and preventing impairment of their health and development. The Children Act 2004 provides the legal framework for the Every Child Matters (ECM) programme for change (DfES 2003), which focuses on improving the 'five outcomes' for all children, that is, not just those in need, or at risk of significant harm. These five outcomes are outlined in the ECM and reiterated in the Children Act 2004 and are described as follows: be healthy; stay safe; enjoy and achieve; make a positive contribution; and achieve economic well-being.

Take some time to review the definition of safeguarding children and the five ECM outcomes and think about what a child needs to optimize their life chances. Describe how these needs might be met and who you think might be responsible for meeting them. Here are some suggestions that you might like to consider along with your own:

- physical needs – food, shelter, somewhere to sleep and play safely. Access to medical services;
- emotional needs – loving parent(s)/carer(s) who can respond to the emotional needs of their child. This will include comfort, praise and setting boundaries to give the child confidence;
- social needs: friends and family in order to develop relationships and to understand their place in the world and how the world works.

Can you identify services and organizations that support families in meeting these needs?

As we saw in Chapter 2, the structure and role of community has changed considerably within recent decades and has subsequently impacted on the way society safeguards and protects its children. In the past, the extended family and community had a significant role in supporting child rearing but would also deal with abusive parents. But as families have become more fragmented through geographical distance because of employment or divorce, for example, the state has become responsible for the regulation of safeguarding and child protection systems (Munro 2010). This also includes the regulation of individuals working with children. The ISA (2009), which has historically set out criteria for anyone working with vulnerable groups, is currently reviewing this process. Up to date information about the process is available at http://www.isa.homeoffice.gov.uk/.

In 2004, as part of the Children Act, Local Safeguarding Boards (LSCB) were set up so that organizations that work with children, whether in the private, voluntary or public sector, would work more closely and in a more streamlined way to safeguard children. Each organization will identify Safeguarding Leads, to support staff and to educate individuals about their role in safeguarding and to give advice about the processes which need to be put in place to ensure that everyone is aware of the safeguarding procedures.

Children's Trusts were also established so that all organizations with responsibilities for children might come together under one umbrella to streamline the coordination of service commissioning for their locality. The fundamental principle of this shift was to remove the barriers between agencies so that those families requiring support receive this at an earlier point and are prevented from becoming child protection cases.

The agencies that are represented within these Trusts include health, education, local authorities, local council, and the voluntary and private sectors.

Health visitors and school nurses have a key function in safeguarding and child protection and work closely with families and other agencies to promote the well-being of children. The health visitor and school nurse's relationship with a family is unique. Health visitors and school nurses have special access to families during health and development checks that other professionals do not (Healthy Child Programme, DH 2008). The unique position of both these professional groups should allow them to be influential and key players in child-protection surveillance. Health visitors and school nurses have no statutory responsibility for child protection. However, they are involved in the interagency consultations that occur when there is a referral to social services.

Childhood has been viewed differently across the centuries and there is plenty of evidence to show that child abuse is not a new phenomenon. Indeed, Charles Dickens gives a very vivid account of the appalling conditions and treatment of young children in his novels *Oliver Twist* and *David Copperfield*. What has changed, however, is our perspective of childhood and the importance and value we place on children and their welfare. One of the key tenets of our society in the twenty-first century is that children and young people have a right to be safeguarded from harm in order to achieve 'optimum life chances and enter adulthood successfully'. Indeed, in 1989 the United Nations Convention on the Rights of the Child set out some principles and standards for the treatment and care of children. Article 19 focuses on issues pertaining to child abuse:

> State parties shall take all appropriate legislative, administrative, social and educational measures to protect the child from all forms of physical or mental violence, injury or abuse, neglect or negligent treatment, maltreatment or exploitation, including sexual abuse, while in the care of parent(s), legal guardians or any other persons who have legal care of the child.
>
> (United Nations 1989: 318)

Child protection therefore refers to a range of activities that are undertaken by individuals and organizations to protect identified children who are experiencing or likely to experience significant harm. Child protection is an essential component of safeguarding and promoting the welfare of children and involves the parents, child and extended family and individuals working within health, education, social services, the police and private and voluntary organizations. What is key to protecting children is the ability of all interested parties to work together to achieve this goal. The 2006 document, *Working Together to Safeguard Children* (DfES 2006b) clearly stresses that communication, sharing of concerns and clear referrals between the involved parties not only protects the child but supports the components of well-being in the 2004 Children Act (2004, Section 10(2), pp. 7–8).

Let's consider Mary's situation and how the principles of safeguarding and child protection have been utilized to support the family through some significant difficulties.

Mary has become increasingly concerned over recent months about her safety and that of her boys, as a friend has informed her that her ex-partner Paul has been released from prison and wants contact with Peter and Simon. Paul is now living in a town ten miles away but has relatives who live in Chettlesbridge.

Mary has been visited by the health visitor, who has referred Mary to the social worker and a police officer from the Domestic Violence Team. The social worker has visited and Mary is now seeking legal advice about how to ensure that her ex-partner is prevented from visiting the home or local vicinity.

Mary left Paul after a very difficult violent relationship, to move back in with her mother. Mary has worked very hard to rebuild her life so that she can give the care the boys need. Before Paul was sentenced, the courts had served an injunction on him which prevented him having contact with Mary or the boys on his release.

Peter and Simon were placed on the Child Protection register a few months after they were born, as Mary had become very depressed and was unable to meet the boys' physical and emotional needs and protect them from significant harm.

The boys began to lose weight and developed repeated bouts of diarrhoea and infective nappy rash. The health visitor had been visiting the family regularly and discussed her concerns about the twins with Mary and the GP. It was agreed that a referral was made to the community paediatrician. Mary had been advised to seek support for her depression but was reluctant.

A week later, Peter was admitted to hospital for dehydration after another bout of diarrhoea. On examination, Peter was discovered to have bruising consistent with deliberate pinching of the tops of his arms. It was at this point that Mary disclosed the violent relationship and her partner's rough handling of Peter and a referral was made to social services. The situation had become a case of suspected child abuse and a case conference was called.

 Reflection

The World Health Organization defined child abuse as: 'all forms of physical and/or emotional ill-treatment, sexual abuse, neglect or negligent treatment or commercial or other exploitation, resulting in actual or potential harm to the child's health, survival, development or dignity in the context of responsibility, trust or power.

(WHO 1999: 13–17)

If we consider the WHO definition, can you describe the grounds for the referral to social services?

In this case, you would be right to think that the family were referred to social services because of the bruising which indicated that Peter had been physically abused. Physical abuse may involve 'hitting, shaking, throwing, poisoning, burning or scalding, drowning, suffocating, or otherwise causing physical harm to a child' (Munro 2010: 49). However, concerns were also raised about Mary's care of the boys which was considered to be neglectful. It was clear that Mary was under enormous stress and very depressed, but concerns were raised about her ability to protect her children.

Neglect is described as:

> the persistent failure to meet a child's basic physical and psychological needs, likely to result in the serious impairment of the child's health or development. It may involve a parent or carer failing to provide adequate food, shelter or clothing, failing to protect a child from physical danger or harm, or failing to ensure access to appropriate medical care or treatment. It may also include neglect of a child's basic emotional needs.
>
> (Turney and Turner 2005: page 3)

There are two other main categories of abuse: sexual abuse, which

> involves forcing or enticing a child or young person to take part in sexual activities, whether or not the child is aware of what is happening. The activities may involve physical contact, including penetrative or non penetrative acts. They may include non contact activities, such as involving children in looking at pornographic material or watching sexual activities, or encouraging children to behave in sexually inappropriate ways.
>
> (Munro 2010: page 49)

The other is emotional abuse, which 'is the persistent emotional ill-treatment of a child such as to cause severe and persistent adverse effects on the child's emotional development. It may involve conveying to children that they are worthless or unloved, inadequate or valued only in so far as they meet the needs of another person' (Munro 2010: 49).

Mary's mother Eileen was very upset as she and Mary had had a very good relationship until Mary moved in with Paul. Eileen had not had contact with her daughter for months and had been very concerned for Mary's welfare.

Common Assessment Framework

Mary's case is undoubtedly very complex and it is in such cases that the Common Assessment Framework (CAF; DfES 2006a) (see Chapter 5) process enables the different agencies to work in a coordinated way to meet children's needs and protect them from harm. The CAF focuses on three key areas which include the child's developmental needs, the parents' capacity and ability to respond to these needs, and the potential and capacity of the extended family and environment to support the child.

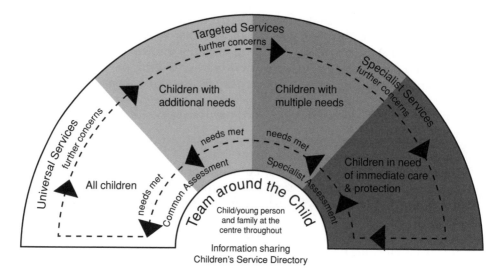

**Continuum of Needs
(commonly known as The Windscreen)**

Figure 4.1 Common Assessment Framework
Source: DfES (2006a)

Figure 4.1 demonstrates how children with different needs are supported. Mary's twins immediately came under the final section of children in need and of immediate care and protection.

Once a child protection team receives a referral, a decision must be made within one working day about what action needs to be taken. The team has a duty to investigate the concerns. If the decision is taken that the child may be at risk, an initial assessment is necessary to gather more information. This initial assessment must be completed within ten working days of the referral to the child protection team (DCSF 2009).

In this case the child protection team considered the boys to be at significant harm.

Case scenario

A case conference was called and Mary and Eileen both attended. Information had been gathered from the health visitor, GP, paediatric consultant, Police, Social Services and education. At the end of the conference the twins were placed on the Child Protection Risk register for physical abuse.

If we review the CAF model, what becomes clear is that a plan has to be put in place so that children's needs are met and in the case of Mary's twins, the agencies involved need to ensure that any plan will protect children from further harm. A key worker will be nominated to lead the child protection process and a series of review meetings will take place to monitor and assess progress and review support and identify further need.

This is the plan that was put in place for the family:

- *Mary would move back to live with her mother in order to remove herself and the twins from Paul.*
- *Paul was to have no contact with Mary or the twins and the police and domestic violence team would be working with Mary and Eileen to ensure that alert systems were in place should Paul make contact.*
- *Mary had agreed to see the GP and a counsellor at the medical practice to help her with her depression.*
- *The health visitor would undertake regular visits to the family home to monitor the twins' growth and development and to support Mary with parenting.*
- *Mary would be referred to a parenting support group at the Limestreet Children's Centre.*
- *The social worker would undertake regular visits to assess the family's progress and assess the continued risk to the twins.*
- *The community paediatrician would undertake further clinical assessments to monitor the twins.*
- *The social worker was identified as keyworker for the family and would ensure that the processes to protect the twins and meet their needs were put in place.*

The outcome of the referral and placing the children on the Child Protection Register, although initially very difficult for Mary, enabled her to accept support and help to focus on the care of the twins. Eileen was able to support Mary emotionally and practically and within a few months of the initial case conference Mary was less depressed and the twins appeared to be thriving.

A series of review meetings took place and because of the significant improvement in Mary and her ability to protect and provide for her twins the twins were removed from the register. Support from the social worker, health visitor and the Children's Centre has continued up until Mary's recent concerns.

 Reflection

Consider the plan that was put in place for the family.

- What are the issues for Mary and her twins now?
- Who and how can she be supported to continue to care for and protect her twins?

Chapter summary

This chapter is about the different elements of protecting people from harm; whether it be disease or environmental disaster; or whether it be physical or emotional abuse of an adult or child. All of these areas are complex and demand an inter-professional approach and common language so risk is managed and protection ensured. As a student it is unlikely that you will become involved in some of the activities discussed in this chapter; however you need to be aware of the systems that protect the population so that if you have concerns you can refer appropriately.

NMC Essential Skill Cluster (ESC)	ESC number
Care, Compassion and Communication	1, 3, 4, 5, 7
Organizational Aspects of Care	9, 12, 15
Infection Prevention and Control	27, 28
Nutrition and Fluid Management	

References

Action on Elder Abuse (2006) *What is Elder Abuse?* http://www.elderabuse.org.uk/About%20Abuse/What_is_abuse%20define.htm (accessed 23 March 2011).

Association of Social Services Directors (2005) *Safeguarding Adults: A National Framework of Standards for Good Practice and Outcomes in Protecting Adults.*

Barker, R. (ed.) (2009) *Making Sense of Every Child Matters: Multi-professional Practice Guidance.* Bristol: The Policy Press.

Brown, K. (2010) *Vulnerable Adults and Community Care.* Exeter: Learning Matters.

Care Quality Commission (2010) *Essential Standards of Quality and Safety.* Care Quality Commission.

Day, R., Bantry-White, E. and Glavin, P. (2010) Protection of vulnerable adults: an interdisciplinary workshop. *Community Practitioner*, 83(9): 23–32.

Department for Education and Skills (DfES) (2003) *Every Child Matters.* London: DfES.

DfES (2006a) *The Common Assessment Framework for Children and Young People: Practitioners' Guide.* London: DfES.

DfES (2006b) *Working Together to Safeguard Children: A Guide to Inter-agency Working to Safeguard and Promote the Welfare of Children.* London: DfES.

Department of Education (2010) *Children in Need in England, Including their Characteristics and Further Information on Children who were Subject of a Child Protection Plan (Children in Need Census) Year Ending March 2010.* London: Department of Education.

DH (Department of Health) (1998) *Modernising Social Services.* London: DH.

DH (2000) *No Secrets: Guidance on Developing and Implementing Multi-agency Policies and Procedures to Protect Vulnerable Adults from Abuse.* London: DH.

DH (2003) *The Victoria Climbie Inquiry: Report of an Inquiry by Lord Laming.* London: HMSO.

DH (2008) *Health and Social Care Act.* London: HMSO.

DH (2009) *Safeguarding Adults: Report on the Consultation on the Review of No Secrets.* London: DH.

DH (2010) *Clinical Governance and Adult Safeguarding: An Integrated Process.* London: HMSO.

DH (2011) *Safeguarding Adults: The Role of Health Service Practitioners.* London: DH.

DCSF (Department for Children, Schools and Families) (2009) *The Protection of Children in England: A Progress Report.* London: HMSO.

Griffiths, R. and Tengnah, C. (2009) Understanding the Safeguarding Vulnerable Groups Act 2006. *British Journal of Community Nursing,* 14(7): 309–13.

Independent Safeguarding Authority (2009) *ISA Referral Guidance.* http://www.isa-gov.org.uk/PDF/ISA%20Referral%20Guidance%20%20V2009-02.pdf (accessed March 2011).

Kim, J. (2009) Type-specific intergenerational transmission of neglectful and physically abusive parenting behaviour among young parents. *Children and Youth Services Review,* 31(7): 761–7.

Lazenbatt, A. (2010) *The Impact of Abuse and Neglect on the Health and Mental Health of Children and Young People.* London: NSPCC.

Mansell, J., Beadle Brown, J., Cambridge, P., Milne, A. and Whelton, B. (2009) Adult protection incidence of referrals, nature and risk factors in two English authorities. *Journal of Social Work,* 9: 23–38.

Milne, A. (2011) Commentary on protecting my mother. *The Journal of Adult Protection,* 13(1): 53–6.

Munro, E. (2010) *Effective Child Protection,* 2nd edn. London: Sage.

NMC (Nursing Midwifery Council) (2008) *The Code: Standards of Conduct, Performance and Ethics for Nurses and Midwives.* London: NMC.

NMC (2010) *Essential Skills Clusters and Guidance for their Use.* London: Nursing Midwifery Council.

O'Keefe, M., Hills, A., Doyle, M. et al. (2007) *UK Study of Abuse and Neglect of Older People Prevalence Survey Report.* London: National Centre for Social Research Kings College.

Pinkney, L., Penhale, B., Manthorpe, J. et al. (2008) Voices from the frontline: social work practitioners' perceptions of multi-agency-working in adult protection in England and Wales. *Journal of Adult Protection,* 10(4): 12–24.

Rees, K. (2011) Protecting my mother, *The Journal of Adult Protection,* 13(1): 46–52.

Turney, D. and Turner, K. (2005) Understanding and working with neglect. *Research in Practice: Every Child Matters Research Briefings,* 10: 1–8.

United Nations (1989) *The United Nations Convention on the Rights of the Child.* New York: United Nations.

World Health Organization (1999) *Report of the Consultation on Child Abuse Prevention, Social Change and Mental Health, Violence and Injury Prevention.* Geneva: World Health Organization. http://www.yesican.org/definitions/WHO.html

World Health Organization (2011) *Elder Abuse.* http://www.who.int/ageing/projects/elder_abuse/en/ (accessed 29 March 2011).

Useful websites

Care Quality Commission www.cqc.org.uk
Every Child Matters www.education.gov.uk
Healthy Child Programme www.dh.gov.uk
Independent Safeguarding Authority www.isa-gov.org.uk
Working Together to Safeguard Children www.education.gov.uk

5 Working with others in community settings

Introduction

This chapter aims to explore working with others in community settings. Effective communication in the assessment, planning and delivery of community nursing care to patients and clients is explored within the context of collaborative, inter-professional working and primary care settings including 'the third sector' (defined by the Charity Commission (2004) as charitable and voluntary organizations). Patient autonomy and inter-professional and collaborative working are aspects of community care that contribute to quality community nursing care delivery.

Chapter 6 explores in more depth the impact of nursing interventions on health. In order to manage differing priorities and resources in the community to meet the needs of patients in their own home environments, the community nurse will be drawing upon their skills to be patient centred. At the same time, community nurses must understand the importance of risk management, the need to prioritize care based on a health needs assessment and the need to work inter-professionally and collaboratively with others within the health and social care arena (the public sphere) and the need to work with patients, families, friends and carers and the third sector (the private sphere).

Some health and social care organizations have, following a risk management analysis, introduced a new framework for working in the community, which is commonly referred to as The Common Assessment Framework (CAF). It is designed to facilitate a patient-centred approach with one key worker drawn from either health (as in a community nurse) or social services or the third sector (an example would be Home-Start, working with families under 5 years, or Age Concern working with older people) who takes the lead in working with patients and their carers and families. The purpose is to improve communication between service users and service providers and to use a common means of communication through a common assessment framework, clear pathways, shared documentation and record keeping and therefore professional accountability and transparent decision making and assessment. White et al. (2009) argue that 'the CAF is a needs-led, evidence-based tool which will promote uniformity, ensure appropriate "early intervention", reduce referral rates . . . and lead to the evolution of a "common language" amongst . . . professionals' (2009: 1).

Learning outcomes

At the end of this chapter you should be able to:

- understand the importance of communication and collaboration for effective patient care in the community;
- recognize the potential barriers to effective working with others in community settings and potential solutions to minimize the barriers and maximize a patient-centred approach to community care delivery.

As a community nurse, it is vital to recognize the 'real world' of community nursing which involves the reflection of legal, professional and ethical frameworks of community nursing care. Schön (1983) was influential in examining how professional knowledge is expanded with reflection-in-action: reflection should be at the centre of an understanding of what professionals do. Sometimes this is referred to as 'thinking on our feet'. Schön argues this involves professionals (as an example of a body of people) to look to their experiences, to connect with their feelings and to attend to the theories that the professionals use in their work (http://www.infed.org/thinkers/et_schon.htm).

An example would be the principles of infection control as a body of knowledge acquired by the community nurse which may conflict with the patient's chosen lifestyle and the patient's home environment. For example, undertaking a wound assessment in a client's home, there maybe numerous free ranging animals impacting on personal hygiene and aseptic techniques but the client wishes to maintain this lifestyle in their own home. Community nurses are guided by the NMC Code of Conduct (2008b) which clearly states individuals' wishes must be respected. The guiding principles therefore underpinning assessing and decision making in community nursing is patient choice, consent, evidence-based care, dignity and respect. Central to those principles is clarity of communication, written, verbal and non-verbal.

Communication

 Questions

Ask yourself the following and write down your answers.

- Can you define the term communication?
- Can you list the types of communication you will use as a community nurse?
- Can you list the means of communication your patients and the patients' carers will use to communicate with you and others?
- Can you identify the rationale for effective communication? Will your rationale be the same as your patient and or their family/carer or friend?
- Will your rationale for effective communication skills be the same as others working in community care, e.g. social services and the third sector?

Reflection

Take a moment to consider your answers – was it easy to define communication? How many means of communication have you identified? Were your answers based on your personal experience or have you also drawn on your experiences as a student nurse? Does it matter if we take only a personal view or should we also be focusing on the patient's experience in developing emotional intelligence and empathy to be effective communicators?

It would be useful to consider the following definitions when exploring communication skills:

- **Communication** refers to the reciprocal and effective process in which messages are sent and received between two or more people (Bach and Grant 2011).
- **Empathy** is the ability to be attuned, and respond appropriately, to the inner experience and distress of patients and clients (Bach and Grant 2011).
- **Experiential learning** is learning that is derived from or relating to experience, as opposed to other methods of acquiring knowledge (Bach and Grant 2011).
- **Emotional intelligence (EI)** is the ability to use one's own and others' emotions effectively for solving problems and living happily (Gardner 2000). Goleman (1998) identifies five domains of EI:
  - knowing your emotions;
  - managing your own emotions;
  - motivating yourself;
  - recognizing and understanding other people's emotions;
  - managing relationships, i.e. managing others' emotions.
- **Interpersonal skills** are exhibited when nurses demonstrate their abilities to use evidence-based, and theory-based, styles of communication with their patients/clients and colleagues (Bach and Grant 2011).

Bach and Grant (2011) outline the importance of effective communication and interpersonal skills to nursing as skilful communication with patients makes a positive healing difference to clients and patients. Specifically this includes patients/clients:

- feeling listened to;
- feeling that their concerns are being validated and not trivialized;
- feeling supported;
- feeling understood.

It is argued that the principles of effective communication and communication skills may be applied equally in all settings and with all others. Some of these issues will be explored further in Chapters 6 and 10.

Professional codes of practice and rules of social engagement

There are professional codes of practice (e.g. NMC 2008b) which guide degrees of intimacy between professionals and patients/carers who are in turn informed by legal, statutory and professional roles and responsibilities.

There are also 'rules of social engagement' (Bach and Grant 2011: 71) which guide how we should behave both as individuals and professionals. Social rules govern or guide how we behave – these evolve from our experience of family and social groups (Bach and Grant 2011). Professional behaviour we learn from experience, role modelling and understanding the application of theory to practice.

 Questions

Do all health and social care professionals share the same codes of conduct? Is the third sector answerable to the same codes of conduct?

Take a moment to access the websites listed at the end of this chapter for the codes of practice guiding health and social care professionals like nurses, social workers and doctors.

Do they share the same values and responsibilities and accountability? Could the differences in codes facilitate or hinder effective communication between professionals and the third sector? Do patients and carers themselves have access to these codes of conduct and therefore will use these in their communication with you? The websites are in the public domain and therefore patients and carers are able to read and make judgements themselves.

 Reflection

Look back at your answers to the questions on page 76. You will probably have cited the spoken word or language. Factors to consider therefore are the language(s) spoken by the client/patient and age of the client/patient.

There are a range of roles undertaken by community nurses where excellent communication skills are needed to practise. A school nurse will be communicating with both primary school aged children or secondary school students, i.e. teenagers: both groups will have different levels of spoken language and communication expertise and skills which you will need to understand. Health visitors may be liaising with a carer whose first language is not English, for example an asylum seeker with a baby. A district nurse may be communicating with an elderly person who is hard of hearing.

Bach and Grant (2011) identify that some nurses demonstrate a lack of respect with elderly nursing home residents by using 'baby talk' and related voice tone and parental style. This example indicates that it is not just the spoken word that is important but also the tone and pitch as well as the appropriateness of the spoken word.

Consider Larry and Michael. As a community nurse you may be communicating with Michael who is distressed that his brother Larry is going to leave him home alone as he is going into hospital – at least that is his perception and it is making him angry. Your effectiveness as a communicator depends on your ability to respond with empathy and professionally to a variety of emotions as well as having unique skills in communicating with people with learning disabilities.

Communication between all people is very complex: miscommunication may lead to misunderstandings, confusion and indeed conflict. This is a particular challenge when working with people with communication needs to ensure that they receive the highest quality of person-centred support (http://www.normanmark.net). Many people with learning disabilities have some difficulties with communication; this may be in understanding what other people are 'saying' or in expressing themselves to others. Examples would be difficulties understanding abstract concepts and in interpreting language, tone of voice, facial expression and body language. There are also issues in sending messages – many factors contribute to the difficulties people with learning disabilities have in enabling others to understand them. For example they make lack the words to express themselves or find it difficult to articulate meanings. They may use the right words but in the wrong order or without the appropriate body language. As a community nurse, you will need to ensure that you are communicating in a way that the person understands. This may include using simple, short sentences and trying to avoid language that will lead to confusion or misunderstanding. Objects, pictures and symbols are particularly useful as ways of reminding people what will be occurring throughout their day (anticipation of events is particularly important) and of supplementing spoken language, as is signed communication (Challenging Behaviour Foundation, http://www.challengingbehaviour.org.uk).

Therapists working with adults with learning disabilities aim to promote communication skills for independence, choice, inclusion and rights. Certain scenarios such as medical treatment can be a barrier to communication for a person with learning disabilities as they may find the scenario stressful, which in turn makes it difficult for them to communicate with others (www.helpwithtalking.com/speech-issues/learning-disability). Your inter-professional working with Michael's social worker is vital to ensure that communication is patient centred and needs led.

You may also have identified non-verbal communication in your reflections. This is an overarching term to include all communication that is not verbal and it is very much centred on body language, facial expressions and body energy and movement. It is argued that 7 per cent of communication is verbal communication, 38 per cent is vocal (volume, pitch, rhythm, etc.) and 55 per cent is body movements (mostly facial expressions) (Barbour and Mele 1976). You may have noted also that non-verbal communication includes the types of clothes we wear, how we dress our hair, how we apply make-up, tattoos and so on. In some cultures, symbols are effective ways of communicating meaning and do not require a spoken word. This is particularly relevant when nurses are assessing pain or anger to avoid conflict such as with Michael.

The legal principle of capacity to consent to and refuse medical treatment must guide all medical procedures. In most cases health professionals cannot legally examine or treat any adult without his or her valid consent. 'Medical procedures' means examination, diagnostic tests and medical or nursing interventions aimed at alleviating a medical condition or preventing its deterioration (British Medical Association and the Law Society 2004). Capacity is the ability to make decisions about a particular matter at a particular time: the legal definition of people who lack capacity is in Section 2 of the Mental Capacity Act 2005 (Dimond 2008). Age Concern (Capacity and Consent: Policy Position Papers accessed www.nmc-uk.org/Documents/Safeguarding/England) states that everyone makes decisions and it is a basic human right to be able to express one's opinion. Individual decisions are often influenced by belief systems, values and ethical considerations including the perception of quality of life. Ageism and stereotypical thinking by others and the person themselves may well influence decisions made. Age Concern continues that the law presumes that every adult has the capacity (or is 'competent') to make his or her own decisions when they have a choice, the necessary tools (like time and information) and understanding with which to decide unless the contrary is established). It is important that a community nurse understands that consent is demonstrated when an individual (either verbally or non-verbally) indicates what they are willing to do or allow a third party to do to or for them. To give valid consent, people need to be able to access, understand and process information relating to the decision they are making and sometimes they may not agree with the community nurse. This means that the community nurse has to respect others' decision making if they are clear that the person has made a decision based on an informed choice and because they have the capacity to make that decision. Age Concern (2011: 1) clarifies further: 'informed consent is therefore a fundamental aspect of any form of health or social care. The mental capacity of an individual is the centre of issues relating to consent'.

The nurse's uniform as a symbol of non-verbal communication

Uniforms are a pertinent symbol that we can draw upon to illustrate non-verbal communication as a means of telling/informing another person a narrative without verbal communication.

Indeed nurses have uniform policies to standardize their working attire – it is argued that this is part of their professional identity.

Questions

Is a uniform policy applied to all others working with clients/patients in the community? What is the purpose of a uniform? What is the message of a nurse in uniform?

You may have considered:

- a uniform as a means of communication;
- a uniform sends out a clear message of professionalism;
- crucial to the uniform is a name badge or personal Identification (ID).

Discussion point

Make a list of the positive and possible negative aspects of a nurse's uniform when considering communication in the community. Discuss with your mentor and colleagues. It would be useful for you to share your reflections with community nurses working in the community care settings. It would also be beneficial to access your Trust Policy on Uniform Attire to enable you to formulate an informed opinion on the role of uniforms in community nursing.

Written communication

One means of communication you may have considered in your reflections so far is written communication. Written communication in community nursing practice requires skill – it must be clear, accurately reflect what took place and be contemporaneous. Therefore written communication is guided by professional, legal and ethical frameworks and may only be recorded in appropriate documents (NMC 2008a).

The purpose of clear accurate and contemporaneous record keeping is to ensure smooth communication between professionals, others and patients and their carers. This is to minimize risk and to allow a mechanism by which all information is accurately transcribed. Other factors which guide accurate written communication are confidentiality (NMC 2008a).

The CAF is one practice example where there has been an attempt to be patient centred and improve written communication by sharing a common assessment and common documentation (White et al. 2009).

Another factor to be mindful of as a community nurse is patient-held records. District nurses in the main keep patient records in the home environment to facilitate communication between professionals. However, other professionals may not be so open in their record keeping as they do not want to share information with a carer or patient – you should bear in mind that every patient has the right to access their record (NMC 2008a).

The storage and written recordings of patient contacts may vary according to the service provider. This may be confusing for patients and professionals alike and may lead to duplication of records. Some record keeping requires IT skills, e.g. the practice nurse may only record patient records electronically. Thus there may be a multitude of examples of recording written information. The author of Chapter 3 explores in more depth the practicalities of working as a community nurse.

Another purpose of clear record keeping is direction finding for other providers of care. Therefore clear note taking of address/contact details are essential particularly for the first contact with the community nurse. It may be that the initial contact is via telephone contact. Student nurses should seek guidance in how to 'take a telephone message' as each employer may have their own written standards. Taking accurate and timely telephone messages is a vital part of a community nurse's communication activities. Many community nurses' offices operate a voice mail or answer machine for taking messages in their absence. There will be a 'message book' for telephone calls that others may use – again you will need to seek guidance on the correct recording of messages. There will be a minimum standard including date, time of message, who the message is for, content of the message and lastly a section where the recipient of the message records that they have received the message. It is also important to be aware of mobile telephone communication and viable 'signal networks'– this was explored in Chapter 3, which discussed the practicalities of working as a community nurse, particularly under 'lone working' and keeping safe in the community. There may be rules and regulations regarding the use of mobile phones in the community. As a student community nurse you should familiarize yourself with them as it is not acceptable to text/mobile phone while on duty as this may breach Trust policy and guidelines on confidentiality (it would be pertinent to access these policies in order to familiarize yourself with the employee's roles and responsibilities in maintaining confidentiality and to check your understanding of the contract of employment for a registered nurse) and you should ensure that you understand the principles of confidentiality outlined in the NMC Code of Conduct (2008b).

Community nurses may well be issued with Trust mobile phones for work-based activities – again there will be rules and regulations regarding their use and you should discuss mobile phones as a means of communication with the registered community nurse.

Information technology

Information technology (IT) plays an increasingly important role in the means of communication and for recording patient information and data. Some employers require community nurses to complete accurate record keeping with the use of hand held devices. This information forms the basis of epidemiology and health needs assessments and profiling in the community. Indeed all information gathering is used to underpin resource decisions. IT is part of 'real world' of community care nursing. Another aspect of IT is the internet as a means of transmitting information through electronic mail and acquiring information through search engines. Intranet and Internet websites are all tools and means of communication that patients, carers and community workers use. Significantly, recent reports have highlighted that the Internet is a vital means of communication for housebound clients/patients and also for carers. Social networking sites are seen as an effective communication tool in combating social isolation and improving knowledge transfer. However, it is advisable to check that information is not confidential and that consent is sought from all those involved in any forms of communication.

Consider the Chettlesbridge residents Larry and Michael. Internet access would be of benefit to the brothers and indeed all residents in the community. Of course, the brothers are dependent on whether there is an Internet or Broadband facility in their location plus the two brothers will need to have set up an account and own a computer themselves.

However, if the brothers do not have the Internet or a computer, where would you as a community nurse be able to 'sign post' them to a free point of access to the Internet? This type of information is part of the local network/profile that a community nurse should be able to share with their clients Larry and Michael. It would be part of the intelligence of their local community. The obvious location of free access to the Internet and a computer is the library although in the present economic climate such community facilities are under real threat of closure. If this is the case, the community nurse would need to ensure that the profile is updated – linking in with the third sector would be an example of community nurses working collaboratively with others to identify if this arena of practice has another source of either free access to the Internet or subsidized access to the Internet. This is an example of community nurses working creatively – in some locations it is the local pub that offers an Internet service. This is not to be confused with Wi-Fi where the user has to have their own computer to access the system and it can be costly.

If we return to the two brothers Larry and Michael we can see how Larry may find the Internet a very useful tool to learn more about his heart condition but also there may be a website that both Michael and Larry may search to help them problem solve any issues that arise due to Michael's learning difficulties. For example, they both may require information on Statutory Benefits such as Carer's allowance. Or there may be a specific website or blog they can access to facilitate social communication and improve their knowledge about a range of resources that would help make their day to day activities more meaningful. Sometimes the local gardening group set up their own blogs or websites – again this may be intelligence that the community nurse may share or they may signpost them to the third sector who will be able to outline what is relevant to them to improve their quality of life in their community.

Social and health care professionals may offer to email the two brothers if they find that this form of communication is beneficial. Increasingly email to patients/clients is the means of communication many prefer. As the community nurse you may well be using email to communicate with patients, carers and others in the collaborative arena of care delivery. It is important that you are aware of email etiquette and standards in all client/patient information.

Collaborative working and inter-professional working with health and social care and the third sector

A fundamental component of community nursing care is understanding the roles and responsibilities of others working with patients as well as meeting the needs of patients in their own environments. As a community nurse you will be drawing upon your skills to be patient centred as well as responding to the needs of family, friends and carers. We have already shown that a basic essential skill in community nursing is the ability to communicate effectively drawing upon verbal and non-verbal communication skills together with effective report writing and documentation of community nursing assessment and decision making in delivering community nursing care.

We now need to explore the concepts of collaborative working and inter-professional working. This is important as the community landscape is a complex one where there is a variety of expertise both professional and in the third sector. The community nurse is required to have a working knowledge of inter-professional care and delivery and collaboration as a key part of their role is to work across social and health care sectors and boundaries as well as the third sector (which is often characterized by unwaged work but may well be the sole providers of community care).The challenge for community nurses is to work effectively in all settings, to be patient centred and to facilitate partnerships. Larry and Michael have different needs – they have to communicate with different health and social care professionals. Intelligence gathering by community nurses involves emotional intelligence and empathy.

 Questions

What is it like for Larry and Michael to have to communicate with many different individuals and agencies? Write down your answers.

What do we mean by the term collaborative and inter-professional working? Write down some terms which come to mind.

You might have written down words such as:

- working together;
- partnership working with others (you may have listed others in health and social care and the voluntary sector);
- joint working with others;

- team approach;
- cooperating with others;
- sharing planning of care and decision making in the community;
- shared goals, shared responsibility;
- participation;
- contribution from other health professionals, social care, family, friends, carers, voluntary organizations, charitable organizations;
- meeting together;
- sharing skills and expertise;
- working with patients;
- listening to the views of others;
- multi-professional;
- health and Public sector working;
- unpaid workers working with paid workers.

Values and beliefs

You might have thought about values and beliefs that shape your understanding of inter-professional and collaborative working; the term collaborative working might infer negativity to you as this is a term given to those who cooperate traitorously with an enemy (*The Concise Oxford Dictionary* 2001).

However, the word 'collaborate' is a term positively used to describe joint working on an activity or project (*The Concise Oxford Dictionary* 2001). According to the Oxford Dictionary the word originates from the nineteenth century and is from the Latin 'work together'. Clearly, the term collaborate may be used to describe people working together and has become integrated into the language of health and social policy in the twenty-first century for example:

- *National Service Framework for Older People* (DH 2001a);
- *National Service Framework for Children, Young People and Maternity Services* (DH 2004);
- *Creating a patient-led NHS* (DH 2005);
- *Our Health, Our Care, and Our Say: A New Direction for Community Services* (DH 2006).

Bliss (2008) argues that the value of health and social care professionals working together is not a new concept: the phrase 'partnership working' is also used to describe shared activities. Bliss further argues that the variety of language used within policy documents and literature is one example of the challenge facing professionals as they endeavour to work together and form partnerships.

 Reflection

Go back to the words you used to define collaborative working and inter-professional working. Was this an easy exercise or has it been challenging to identify words that reflect the concept of collaborative inter-professional working?

Bliss (2008) would argue that even for advanced primary care or community nurses, the definition of collaboration and inter-professional working is not easy to describe. This is because for example, the terms 'inter-professional' and 'multi-professional' are often used interchangeably.

Bliss (2008) outlines MacIntosh and McCormack's (2001) clarification of the different processes used to reach a common goal from the multi-professional perspective of health and social care delivery and the inter-professional perspective.

It is useful to examine these perspectives as we consider the two brothers Larry and Michael as clearly their health needs are holistic and therefore will involve many services drawn from the public sector (health and social) as well as the private or third sector (family, friends, carers, voluntary, charitable). The key challenge is how all these services are delivered and if services focus on the client or patient as the central part of assessment and decision making.

It may be useful at this point to define the terms 'multi' and 'inter' as outlined by Bliss (2008):

Multi
Partners from different domains work *independently* to achieve a common purpose.
   Words used to describe these partners would be:

- multidisciplinary
- multi-sectoral
- multi-professional

Inter
Partners from different domains work *interdependently* to achieve a common purpose.
   Words used to describe these partners would be:

- interdisciplinary
- inter-sectoral
- inter-professional

Reflection

It is useful to pause and reflect on the terms

- discipline
- professional
- sectoral

What do these terms mean to you? How are they used in practice?

According to the *Oxford English Dictionary* (2001) the word discipline in this context is:

A branch of knowledge, especially one studied in Higher Education

A profession is:

A paid occupation, especially one involving training and a formal qualification

Professional is:

Of, relating to, or belonging to a profession. Engaged in an activity as a paid occupation rather than as an amateur

A professional person is:

A person having impressive competence in a particular activity

Professionalism is:

The competence or skill expected of a professional, the practising of an activity by professionals rather than amateurs

Sector is:

An area or portion that is distinct from others – a distinctive part of an economy, society, or sphere of activity.

Sectoral is the adjective of the noun sector.

Thus the terms discipline, professional and sector would imply organized conceptual frameworks that are driven by professionals although the term sectoral may include unpaid organizations which are distinct from public funded and paid settings such as health and social care. Did you consider any of these definitions in your reflection?

Defining attributes of collaboration

To be an effective community nurse we must consider the client or patient. We need to focus on them as the centre of any care assessment, planning and delivery. Our community nursing care perspectives must include an understanding of the characteristics of person-centred care.

A good start is to consider the defining attributes of collaboration outlined by Henneman et al. (1995) who argue that the underpinning principle of inter-professional working is that of collaboration but it is a complex phenomenon. As community nurses, a common understanding facilitates effective partnership working. Henneman et al.'s (1995) (see Bliss 2008) defining attributes of collaboration are:

- joint venture;
- willing participation;
- team approach;
- shared responsibility;
- power is shared: based on expertise;
- knowledge and expertise versus role or title;
- cooperative behaviour;
- shared planning and decision making;
- contribution of expertise;
- non-hierarchical relationships.

If we explore the above attributes and apply them to the brothers Larry and Michael, we can see that underpinning all assessment and decision making is person-centred care. Certainly recent policy drivers have recognized patient expertise in the experience of living with and management of long-term conditions. Indeed the Department of Health recognizes the unique skills of the 'expert patient' and advises health and social care professionals to take a new approach when working with patients with long-term conditions through recognizing and utilizing these skills for the benefit of others (DH 2001a, 2001b).

It can be argued that Larry is an expert carer, caring for his brother with learning difficulties. Clearly, Larry's health need and admission to hospital means that he cannot care for his brother. The importance of a partnership approach to planning for Larry to go into hospital and for Michael to continue to be cared for in his home environment will include an inter-professional, inter-sectoral approach.

 Reflection

Think about the two brothers' health and social needs as Larry prepares for his admission to hospital. List the people that will be involved – include professionals as well as non professionals. List the agencies that will be involved – include professional agencies as well as the third sector.

Now consider the organizational aspects of planning the care delivery to the brothers – you may for example consider the leader or coordinator is very important.

Who would this be?

You might be reflecting on patients' rights, patient autonomy and patient choice.

You might identify that there are tensions between identified health needs and the allocation of resources according to priority and cost. You might consider that this case scenarios is an example of collaboration between a range of agencies from public to private. Bliss (2008) argues that collaboration improves the patient experience.

To help you with the above activity, it is useful to explore the characteristics of person-centred care.

The following have been identified as characteristics of person-centred care (DH 2008):

- sharing power and responsibility;
- promoting choice and autonomy;
- promoting inclusion;
- upholding a person's rights;
- keeping clients and families informed and involved in decision making;
- respecting others, treating others with dignity;
- listening, acknowledging and actively responding to needs.

In this contemporary model of patient centredness, the client or patient is moving from a position of 'passive recipient' to 'active participant' in the care process. The balance of power is shifting in the patient–professional relationship to placing the patient at the centre.

Brooker (2003) sets out the following as key to person-centred care:

- valuing people and those who care for them;
- treating people as individuals;
- looking at the world from the perspective of the person;
- a positive social environment that enables the person to experience relative well-being.

Innes et al. (2006) argue that, although the exact term used varies, there is general consensus that person-centred care:

- is service user friendly and family focused;
- promotes independence and autonomy;
- Involves service users choosing from reliable flexible services;
- Tends to be offered by those working with a collaborative/team philosophy.

Go back to your reflection on planning Larry and Michael's care. You may want to revisit the previous chapters and other case scenarios.

Critical thinking

The ability to think critically is a core skill that modern nurses need to develop (Price and Harrington 2010) to improve practice. Community nurses need to think critically to integrate theory to practice and to be successful in managing differing priorities and resources and working within a multi-sectoral setting.

 Questions

What do you think may be the barriers to patient-centred care?
   Write them down.
   You may have considered that barriers may not be obvious or transparent. This may be confusing for clients/carer, families and professionals alike. Barriers may be lack of resources, or conflict, poor communication, lack of trust, lack of ownership, poor leadership and coordination (Bliss 2008).

Hardy et al.'s (2003) six partnership principles are set out by Bliss (2008) as relevant for consideration when assessing the development and sustaining of professional partnerships. In some ways, the six principles are suggesting a problem-solving approach to removing the barriers to person-centred care and collaboration.

They are:

Principle 1: recognize and accept the need for partnership
Principle 2: develop clarity and realism of purpose
Principle 3: ensure commitment and ownership
Principle 4: develop and maintain trust
Principle 5: create clear and robust partnership arrangements
Principle 6: monitor, measure and learn

Thus if we consider the health needs assessment of Larry and Michael in the real world of community nursing (plus the other case scenarios) we need to consider the application of the six principles, which may be summed up as follows:

- It is vital to believe in partnership working.
- You must have clear goals and plans that are realistic and flexible.
- Commitment and ownership by all in the delivery of community care is essential.
- Trust is crucial and involves effective communication.
- Partnership works well if there are clear plans.
- Evaluation of care is linked to health outcomes and the patient's experience.

Chapter summary

Return to the learning outcomes of this chapter and reflect on your activities. This chapter has focused on the following:

- Communication skills in community nursing practice involve a range of activities from verbal and non-verbal skills to written documentation and IT skills.
- Patient-centred care requires active listening, respect and patient/client autonomy.
- Community nursing operates within an inter-professional, multi-sectoral landscape.
- The third sector may be the coordinators of assessment and delivery of care.
- Partnership working is crucial to the promotion of flexible, needs assessed care in the community setting.

NMC Essential Skill Cluster (ESC)	ESC number
Care, Compassion and Communication	1, 2, 3, 4, 5, 6, 7, 8,
Organizational Aspects of Care	9, 10, 13, 16
Infection Prevention and Control	24
Nutrition and Fluid Management	
Medicines Management	40

References

Age Concern (2011) *Capacity and Consent: Policy Position Papers.* www.nmc-uk.org/Documents/Safeguarding/England (accessed 20 October 2011).

Bach, S. and Grant, A. (2011) *Communication and Interpersonal Skills in Nursing,* 2nd edn. Exeter: Learning Matters.

Barbour, A. and Mele, K. (1976) *Louder Than Words: Non Verbal Communication.* Columbus, OH: Merrill.

Bliss, J. (2008) Developing and sustaining professional partnerships. In R. Neno and D. Price (eds) *The Handbook for Advanced Primary Care Nurses.* Maidenhead: Open University Press/McGraw-Hill Education.

British Medical Association and the Law Society (2004) *Assessment of Mental Capacity,* 2nd edn. London: BMJ Books.

Brooker, D. (2003) What is person centred care in dementia? *Reviews in Clinical Gerontology,* 13: 215–22.

Charity Commission (2004) http://www.charity-commission.gov.uk/ourregulatory-activity/default.aspx (accessed 23 January 2012).

DH (Department of Health) (2001a) *National Service Framework for Older People.* London: DH.

DH (2001b) *The Expert Patient: A New Approach to Chronic Disease Management.* London: DH.

DH (2004) *National Service Framework for Children, Young People and Maternity Services.* London: DH.

DH (2005) *Creating a Patient-led NHS.* London: DH.

DH (2006) *Our Health, Our Care, Our Say: A New Direction for Community Services,* Cm6737. London: HMSO.

DH (2008) *Leading Local Change (Darzi Report).* London: DH.

Dimond, B. (2008) *Legal Aspects of Mental Capacity.* Oxford: Blackwell.

Gardner, H. (2000) *Intelligence Reframed: Multiple Intelligences for the 21st Century.* New York: Basic Books.

Goleman, D. (1998) *Working with Emotional Intelligence.* New York: Bantam Books.

Hardy, B., Hudson, B. and Waddington, E. (2003) *Assessing Strategic Partnership: The Partnership Assessment Tool.* Strategic Partnership Taskforce. Leeds: Nuffield Institute for Health/London: Office of the Deputy Prime Minister.

Henneman, E.A., Lee, J.L. and Cohen, J.L. (1995) Collaboration: a concept analysis *Journal of Advanced Nursing,* 21: 103–9.

Innes, A., Macpherson, S. and McCabe, L. (2006) *Promoting Person Centred Care at the Front Line.* http://www.jrf.org.uk/publications/promoting-person-centred-care-front-line (accessed 31 August 2011).

Learning Disability http://www.helpwithtalking.com/speech-issues/learning-disability (accessed 20 October 2011).

NMC (Nursing and Midwifery Council) (2008a) Age Concern: Policy and Position Papers: Capacity and Consent. http://www.nmc-uk.org/Documents/Safeguarding/England (accessed 20 October 2011).

NMC (2008b) *The Code of Conduct for Nurses and Midwives.* London: NMC.

Price, B. and Harrington, A. (2010) *Critical Thinking and Writing for Nursing Students.* Exeter: Learning Matters.

Schön, D. (1983) *The Reflective Practitioner: How Professionals Think in Action.* New York: Basic Books.

White, S., Hall, C. and Peckover, S. (2009) The descriptive tyranny of the Common Assessment Framework: technologies of categorization and professional practice in child welfare. *British Journal of Social Work,* 39(7): 1197–217.

Useful websites

General Medical Council www.gmc-uk.org/about/register_code_of_conduct.asp
General Social Care Council www.gscc.org.uk/codes
Joseph Rowntree Trust www.jrf.org.uk

6 Working with carers and their families

Introduction

Prime Minister Gordon Brown (DH 2008) recognized in *Carers at the Heart of 21st-century Families and Communities* that caring for our relatives and a friend when they are in need is a challenge that the vast majority of us will rise to at some point in our lives. This chapter asks you to consider the huge resource carers provide to our health care and support systems (DH 2008) that is often hidden from society. Carers are unpaid workers who have many responsibilities; at any one time, one in ten people is a carer, the majority of them women (DH 2008). The demands both on health and social care and on carers themselves are greater than ever before (DH 2008: 2)

Carers are individuals with their own aspirations. Alongside their role as carer, they may need support so that they can live healthy and independent lives and pursue a career, an education or social activities (DH 2009).

Carers must receive the recognition and status they deserve (DH 2009). Community nurses are in a unique role to facilitate support to carers and to signpost them to other support systems that may enable a comprehensive carer support network. Community nurses are in a special role as they visit individuals in their own home and they have an understanding of their community and neighbourhoods. Community nurses also work collaboratively with others and therefore have local intelligence which promotes a 'whole-area approach to assessing need' (DH 2009). Indeed carers want more personalized support and greater scope to control and customize services including health care when identifying needs and ensuring prompt access to services (DH 2008) including community nursing.

Learning outcomes

At the end of this chapter you should:

- have an understanding of the roles and responsibilities of carers and how these may impact on their health;
- be able to identify the demographics of carers in England and Wales;
- be able to understand the need to personalize the individual needs of each carer to enable them to manage the twin demands of work and caring responsibilities;

- have an understanding of the policy frameworks which aim to place carers at the heart of twenty-first-century families and communities;
- be able to contextualize working with carers and families within the NMC Code of Conduct for Nurses (NMC 2008b).

The NMC Code of Conduct

The themes raised in this chapter should be read within the context of the *NMC Code of Conduct* (NMC 2008b). Also *Care and Respect Every Time: What You Can Expect from Nurses* (NMC 2008a) provides information for older people and their carers about what they can expect from nurses and how to challenge poor care.

'Nurses play a very important part in the care of older people. Good nursing care can make a difference to your quality of life' (NMC 2008a: 1). In *Care and Respect Every Time: What You Can Expect from Nurses* the NMC outlines:

> the care you should expect in any setting where a nurse is caring for you. There are three things that can make a real difference to the care you receive.
>
> **People** – the nurses who care for you
> **Process** – how nurses care for you
> **Place** – where nurses care for you
>
> (NMC 2008a: 1)

The NMC continues to outline in more depth what they mean by people, process and place.

It is important to be clear that you understand the NMC's guidance as this is particularly pertinent to reflecting on carers as 'the heart of 21st century families and communities' (DH 2008a: 1).

Your role as community nurse is to ensure that 'a caring system' for carers is 'on the side' of the the carer to enable the carer to have 'a life' of their 'own' (DH 2008a: 1).

The NMC (2008a) state that:

> **people** should receive care from capable nurses who:
>
> - Have the knowledge, skills, and desire to provide high standard of care which meets your individual needs
> - Tell their colleagues straight away if they see them providing poor care or behaving in a way that causes you distress
> - Are trustworthy, dependable and are there for you when you need them
> - Show empathy, compassion and kindness.

The NMC continues that 'process' means

> you should receive care that makes you feel valued and treated as an individual, by nurses who

- Listen to what you have to say, taking time to communicate in the way that is best for you
- Find out from you, and others who are important to you, how you want to be cared for
- Provide care in a way that respects your right to privacy and dignity
- Work together with you, and the people who are important to you, by making sure that your wishes are taken into account when decisions are being made.

The NMC writes that 'place' is wherever you receive care from a nurse. The NMC continues that

you should

- Feel you are in safe hands
- Believe that your individual needs are being met in a fair, non-judgemental and respectful way
- Be confident that the nurses and the equipment that you need are available
- Be in no doubt that the nurses are committed to ensuring that a high standard of care is delivered.

(NMC 2008a: 1)

In the context of caring by carers, a community nurse needs to have at the forefront of their care delivery the understanding that the carer may be the patient's advocate and the main communicator with health and social professionals: the carer too deserves and must expect from nurses 'care and respect every time' (NMC 2008a: 1).

Demography: facts and figures

 Question

Take a few moments to reflect on the age profile of carers and the number of carers in England and Wales. What do you think they may be?

Some statistics

The most recent census results available are from the 2001 census.

There are 5.2 million carers in England and Wales (National Statistics Online 2003). There is no average profile of a carer with caring being taken on across all age groups, ethnic groups and geographic locations (DH 2008).

Did this match your estimation? Are you surprised at the number?

Over the next ten years, there will be significant demographic and social changes in Britain presenting major challenges to government and society (DH 2008). Advancing technology and medicine means that people with complex health conditions are surviving longer and have multiple needs. Changing family life, increased numbers of single member households and the geographical dispersion within families may also have an impact on the availability of carers (DH 2008).

Fact: The number of people over 85 in the UK, the age group most likely to need care, is expected to increase by over 50 per cent to 1.9 million over the next decade (Office for National Statistics, cited by DH 2008).

The 2001 census asked for the first time the question about whether people provided unpaid care for a family member or friend and for how many hours. Over 225 000 people provide 50 or more hours of unpaid care per week. More than half of these people are over 55 years. However, there are nearly 80 000 aged 54 years and under. The age group where the largest proportion of people provide care is in the 50s.

More than one in five people aged 50–59 are providing some unpaid care. About one in four (24.6 per cent) are women in this age group compared with 17.9 per cent of men. Many of the people providing care do paid work as well. Of the 15.2 million employees aged 16–74 in full-time work, 1.6 million are providing at least some unpaid care – 144 000 50 or more hours care a week. For full-time workers providing 50 or more hours there is a larger proportion of men.

Of the nearly 2 million people aged 16–74 who are permantly sick or disabled, over a quarter of a million (273 000) provide some unpaid care for other people and 105 000 provide 50 or more hours care (National Statistics Online 2003).

 Question

What are the issues and concerns for carers as they care for their relatives or friends?

Fact: Over 225 000 people providing 50 or more hours of unpaid care per week state that they are not in good health themselves. More than half of the people providing this much care are over the age of 55 years, and it is at these ages that the 'not good health' is highest (National Statistics Online 2003).

Nearly 80 000 people aged 54 years and under providing more than 50 hours of unpaid work per week state their health was not good (National Statistics Online 2003). These facts and figures are very important to community nurses as they provide the evidence for them to value and empathize with the roles and responsibilities of carers. They also enable them to understand that the carers themselves are at risk from added pressure and stress, which may impact on their own health and health needs. Significantly, people in their 50s may have other domestic responsibilities such as teenage children or being grandparents themselves. This means that carers may have multiple caring responsibilities.

Question

What do you think are the issues and concerns identified by carers themselves?
  The list below shows some of the issues identified by carers:
* lack of information and support;
* lack of respite from caring;
* financial worries;
* lack of time for themselves;
* isolation and loneliness;
* worry about who will care when they cannot;
* carers' own health problems;
* lack of recognition of their role and value.

(Hartlepool Carers 2010)

 Question

What do you think are the effects of caring on carers?
  Below is a list of effects on carers. You may have thought of some of these:
* They are worse off since becoming carers.
* Many have to give up work resulting in a drop in income.
* Increased level of charges for services has caused further financial hardship.
* Carers suffer from tiredness and have difficulty sleeping.
* Many suffer from back problems.
* Carers suffer from depression.
* Carers suffer from stress.
* Carers have to cut back on food and essentials.
* Carers cannot afford to go on holiday.
* Carers have cut down on leisure activities and social life.

(Hartlepool Carers 2010)

Consider some of the residents of Chettlesbridge:

* Mrs Brown receives care from her daughter Elizabeth and they pay for a carer to come into the home. They rely too on friends and neighbours to enable Elizabeth to pursue her hobbies and interests.
* Mary and her twin boys rely on Mary's mother's support for caring for the twins while Mary works as a paid carer and takes in ironing to supplement her income.
* When Larry goes into hospital who will care for Michael who depends on Larry as his primary carer?

Reflection

Return to your answers on what the effects of caring are and compare them to Hartlepool Carers' findings – are your reflections similar?

Now apply the issues and concerns to the above Chettlebridge residents. Do you think the issues will vary according to individual needs?

Consider your answers and reflections in the context of the role of the family and recent policy frameworks.

Recent National Policy frameworks

The Report *Commissioning for Carers: An Action Guide for Decision Makers* (DH 2009) states that carers' contribution to care and support is significant in the UK. It is therefore essential that health and social care encourages and supports carers whatever their level, need or entitlement. Crucially professionals need to ensure that the decision to care is a genuine one, and based on informed choice.

The National Carers' Strategy *Carers at the Heart of 21st-century Families and Communities* (DH 2008) sets out what needs to be achieved for carers by 2018, including:

- protecting carers' own mental and physical health;
- giving carers access to the integrated and personalized services they need to support them;
- ensuring that carers enjoy a life of their own.

 Reflection

Take some time to reflect on the three aims of the National Strategy and consider why it is relevant to community nurses to consider the Strategy for Carers.

- You may have reflected that it is important for primary health and social care teams to collaborate in identifying and supporting carers.
- You may have identified the importance of putting the carer at the centre of a comprehensive assessment of need – 'think carer'.
- You may have identified that community nurses have a unique role in protecting carers' own mental and physical health as they have specific skills and knowledge in nursing assessment, care and intervention.

- You may have identified that community nurses possess neighbourhood intelligence including a working knowledge of local voluntary, charitable agencies that provide valuable information and support or respite to carers.
- You may have identified that carers' voices should be listened to when assessing and making decisions about local services including the design of those services to fit the needs of patients. You may have considered how best community nurses may gather information and listen to carers.

Commissioning for Carers: An Action Guide for Decision Makers (DH 2009) provides a model of comprehensive carer support as a tool in analysing a community's performance against the *National Carers Strategy* (DH 2008). This model has arisen from collaboration between a number of carer and improvement agencies who worked together with local providers and commissioners to develop a model of comprehensive carer support (see Figure 6.1). While this model is intended for anyone making commissioning decisions that could affect adult carers, it presents some of the key themes, questions and challenges that are vital to the delivery of effective community nursing care. If we apply the model to community nursing decision making, we can apply the same aims to facilitate an up to date and flexible community nursing assessment for carers and their families.

So the action guide aims to support commissioners in improving outcomes for carers by:

- taking commissioners through the process of assessing need and putting in place provision to support carers;
- outlining key questions and guidance to assist with commissioning;
- explaining the challenges involved and showing how to assess the effectiveness of services.

Reflection

Take some time to reflect on the above aims but substitute community nursing for commissioners. Now look at the model – what have you observed?
    You may have reflected that the model:

- places the carer in the centre;
- advocates carer-led assessment;
- promotes a whole systems or whole area approach to support;

- incorporates the main determinants of health (Dahlgren and Whitehead 1991) or health needs assessment drawing on a range of factors that affect the activities of daily living;
- places carers at the heart of communities and services; and
- reflects the overarching aim of community nursing which is to provide a service based on health needs including the determinants of health.

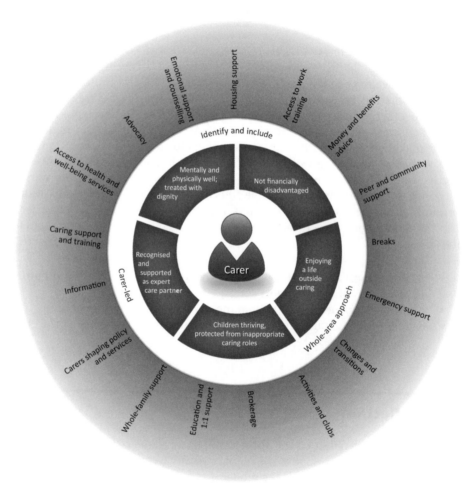

Figure 6.1 A model of comprehensive carer support
(*Source:* Adapted from A Model of Comprehensive Carer Support, Figure 1 (DH 2009). Reproduced with kind permission from The Princess Royal Trust for Carers and Crossroads Care © 2012.

Question

What statutory obligations are there to support carers?

It is important that community nurses have an understanding that carers are entitled to statutory support. All professionals who are in contact with any carer, or who meet new carers, should ensure that the carer is given the option to say what could help them with their caring role (The Princess Royal Trust for Carers 2011). This opportunity may be formalized as a 'Carer's Assessment'. Carers have a legal right to an assessment (The Princess Royal Trust for Carers 2011). It is a statutory obligation for social care and other council staff to undertake a carer's assessment.

 Question

What is the role of the community nurse in statutory carer's assessment?

The role of the community nurse is to ensure that the carer is given the opportunity to be assessed either by referring to social care or signposting the family to social care.

The Princess Royal Trust for Carers (2011) is very clear that if a carer says they do not want an assessment, then the professional needs to find out why. The Trust outlines some reasons for carers refusing an assessment which community nurses must reflect upon:

- The carer may not see the point.
- They do not understand what is on offer to them as carers.
- They don't feel comfortable in talking about their needs (as opposed to those of the person they care for).

The Princess Royal Trust for Carers (2011) is an example of an organization that is not a health or social care agency but rather a charitable organization offering support and lobbying decision makers on behalf of carers. It advises professionals to explain to a carer why a 'formal conversation' about their needs for support is a valuable exercise in assessing their needs for support and not 'a pointless bureaucratic process' (The Princess Royal Trust for Carers 2011: 1).

The Princess Royal Trust for Carers (2011) provides a service to carers. The Trust's vision is that 'Carers are recognised, valued and able to maximise their quality of life'. Their mission is 'To meet the diverse needs of carers through excellent local and national services'. The Princess Royal Trust for Carers (2011) provides further detail around the process of the carer's assessment.

Having a carers assessment allows the carer to:

- look at what help they need to support them as a carer;
- find out what help and support may be available;
- make a decision about the future.

To be eligible for a carer's assessment the carer must:

- be looking after or intending to look after someone who may have community care needs (even if that person has not had a community care assessment or isn't receiving any services); and
- be providing or intending to provide a *substantial amount of care on a regular basis.*

It is important for community nurses to be aware that 'regular' may be once a day or once a month. It does not have a definition in law. The Princess Royal Trust for Carers (2011) is clear that the term 'substantial' depends on the carer's personal circumstances – work or physical ability. It is important to remember that the carer's needs may not match those of the person they care for; for example someone using community services that has moderate needs may have a carer who is experiencing critical need (The Princess Royal Trust for Carers 2011).

 Reflection

Consider our residents of Chettlesbridge – the two brothers Larry and Michael, and Essie and Marvin West (see below).

Take a moment to list voluntary or charitable agencies that may be able to support the carers of these families.

In both families the primary care givers' needs are now critical compared to those they care for in the family (Larry now has a critical need and has to be admitted to hospital for cardiac care; Essie has recently been diagnosed with breast cancer and has three young children).

The community nurse may advise they undergo a carer's assessment as this is a legal right for all carers. However, the community nurses' local Intelligence may also enable them to either refer directly or advise the carer to self refer to local relevant charitable or voluntary agencies.

You may have identified Home-Start for the West family. Home-Start accepts referrals from professionals and also families themselves with children. Home-Start supports 'any family who needs us, as long as they have at least one child under 5' (Home-Start 2011: 1).

Home-Start states the following:

As a parent you might ask for Home-Start's help for all sorts of reasons:

- You may be feeling isolated in your community, have no family nearby and be struggling to make friends
- You may be finding it hard to cope because of your own or child's illness
- You may have been hit hard by the death of a loved one
- You may be really struggling with emotional and physical demands of having twins or triplets – perhaps born into an already large family

The National Strategy for Caring (DH 2008) recognizes the role family plays but also that the challenge we face as a society, and therefore as professionals, is the balancing of the increase in the number of people requiring care and support. This is because the ready availability of those friends and family members, who are either able to, or willing to, provide care and support may not match the growing numbers of people requiring care. In addition there may be a cost factor to the care required. Organizations such as Home-Start provide support fitting into the model of comprehensive carer support (see Figure 6.1). Voluntary and charitable organizations may fill the gap where family is not a possibility and where health and social care services cannot meet all needs.

You may have identified Mencap – the voice of learning disability – as a charitable organization that may provide support to Larry and his friends now that Larry has a critical need (Mencap 2011).

The Princess Royal Trust for Carers (2011) would be another very useful charitable agency.

The importance of community nurses profiling their communities and neighbourhoods

Profiling the local and national charitable and voluntary agencies and organizations in your neighbourhood is an essential process in providing quality care (see Chapter 9 for more in-depth discussion on the link between quality- and evidence-based care).

The Charity Commission (2004) sets out in detail *The Promotion of the Voluntary Sector for the Benefit of the Public*. The Charity Commission have accepted the promotion of the voluntary sector for the benefit of the public as a charitable purpose in its own right. In general terms, they describe the 'voluntary sector' as bodies which are 'Formally constituted, independent of (central and local) government, self governing, not profit distributing, primary non-business and that benefit from voluntarism and that are not political organisations' (2004: 1).

The Charity Commission (2004) further explains that the voluntary sector is an important part of today's economy and has an important role to play in the nation's life:

> The voluntary and community sector has a vital role in society as the nation's 'third sector' working alongside the state and the market. Through its engagement of volunteers, the services it provides and the support it gives to individuals and groups, its contribution to community and civil life is immense, invaluable and irreplaceable.
>
> (2004: 2)

It is vital that community nurses working with carers and their families understand this important role played by the third sector.

Chapter summary

This chapter has explored the recent policy frameworks which aim to place the carer at the heart of twenty-first-century families and communities. It has outlined the demographic profile of carers and established that there is not an average carer. Carers provide unpaid caring but have issues and concerns that arise out of their caring responsibilities which may impact negatively on their own health and economic status.

Carers have a legal right to a carer's assessment to look at what help is available to them. Community nurses have a vital role in facilitating the assessment of carers' support.

A model of comprehensive carer support has been developed in partnership with the Department of Health and carer and improvement agencies to facilitate a whole area or systems approach to providing assessment and support to carers. Personalizing care recognizes the individual needs of each carer (DH 2009). The personalizing approach fits with the aim of community nurses to provide individualized care to people in their neighbourhoods.

The Department of Health advocates the development of 'community capital': people and families become expert care partners.

Community nurses working with carers and families as partners will facilitate greater choice, control and independence for everyone who uses services – having an understanding of the needs of carers is crucial to achieving that aim. It is also essential that all care giving by community nurses is set within the NMC Code of Conduct (NMC 2008b).

NMC Essential Skill Cluster (ESC)	ESC number
Care, Compassion and Communication	1, 2, 3, 4, 5, 6, 7, 8
Organizational Aspects of Care	9, 10, 13, 16
Medicines Management	40

References

Dahlgren, G. and Whitehead, M. (1991) *Policies and Strategies to Promote Social Equity in Health*. Stockholm: Institute of Future Studies.

The Charity Commission (2004) http://www.charity-commission.gov.uk/Publications/rr13.aspx (accessed 16 August 2011).

DH (Department of Health (2008) *Carers at the Heart of 21st-century Families and Communities*. London: DH.

DH (2009) *Commissioning for Carers: An Action Guide for Decision Makers*. London: DH.

Hartlepool Carers (2010) *Caring Together: Contact us for more information on carers*. http://www.hartlepoolcarers.org.uk/carers.asp (accessed 15 August 2011).

Home-Start (2011) *Support and Friendship for Families*. http://www.home-start.org.uk/needsupport/need_support (accessed 15 August 2011).

Mencap (2011) *The Voice of Learning Disability*. http://www.mencap.org.uk/ (accessed 15 August 2011).

National Statistics Online (2003) http://www.statistics.gov.uk/cci/nugget_print.asp (accessed 8 July 2011).

NMC (Nursing and Midwifery Council) (2008a) *Care and Respect Every Time: What you can expect from nurses*. http://www.nmc-uk.org/General-public/Older-people-and-their-carers/Care-and-respect-every-time/ (accessed 15 August 2011).

NMC (2008b) *The Code: Standards of Conduct, Performance and Ethics for Nurses and Midwives*. http://www.nmc-uk.org (accessed 24 January 2012).

The Princess Royal Trust for Carers (2011) http://professionals.carers.org/social-carers-assessment,4377,PP.html (accessed 15 August 2011).

7 Assessing for care

Introduction

This chapter introduces you to assessment in relation to case scenarios 1 and 4 (see Chapter 1) about the residents of Chettlesbridge and asks you to consider the assessment process within the community setting. You will be invited to explore and apply the transferable skills and knowledge base required to the given case scenario. This will help you reflect on community nursing and consider your own solutions.

This chapter will consider:

- the role of assessment;
- the skills and knowledge required to complete individualized assessments in the community setting;
- documentation.

Learning outcomes

At the end of this chapter you should be able to:

- discuss the role of assessment and identification of an individual and/or family's health and social needs within the community setting;
- recognize the skills, theory and concepts that underpin individualized assessment within the home setting;
- identify effective communication and interpersonal skills that will facilitate a comprehensive, therapeutic and person-centred assessment.

Assessment

McIntosh (2006: 299) stated 'There is a wide recognition that assessment by community nurses is central to the provision of high quality care'. Assessment is an ongoing and complex process that requires a plethora of effective skills such as communication, use of intuition, observation, clinical judgement and the ability to reason, problem solve and facilitate decision making. The ability to recognize and incorporate the perspectives of the patient is paramount if we are to pay more than just lip service to partnership and collaborative working. We must promote choice and autonomy and engage people to be involved in their own care planning and decision making.

The therapeutic relationship

Rogers (1951) suggested a therapeutic relationship has three elements: empathy, genuiness and acceptance, which contribute to effective person-centred care. Although others have suggested that other skills and knowledge are required, the three elements are generally accepted as 'core conditions' for this type of relationship to develop. It is pivotal that the relationship is effective if we are to deliver person-centred care and concepts such as emotional intelligence (Goleman 1996) and personal development (Chapman 2006) can support practitioners to do this. Patients must be valued as such and therefore labelling, stereotyping and stigmatization requires challenging if we are to work in partnership with individuals effectively and complete holistic and accurate assessments incorporating unconditional positive regard (Rogers 1951).

 Question

Refer back to case scenario 1 in Chapter 1 involving Evie Brown and her daughter Elizabeth. When considering the 'therapeutic relationship' and what you have read how might you demonstrate your understanding of the terms empathy, genuineness and acceptance in relation to Evie when communicating with her?

You may have considered the following:

Empathy: it is important to attempt to understand Mrs Brown's individual experience and to put to one side any preconceptions or judgements. Explore how Mrs Brown feels and what her thoughts are.

Genuineness: nurses should be aware of their own thoughts and feelings and be able to connect with Mrs Brown as a 'real' person but acknowledging there are boundaries within a therapeutic relationship. Therefore nurses must remain professional and aware of their own thoughts and feelings but be sensitive, tactful and honest.

Acceptance: nurses need to accept Mrs Brown for the person that she is. As professionals we may not like or 'approve' of the choices people make or the lifestyles individuals choose to live by, perhaps because it does not fit into our own personal belief or values system, but we need to accept other people's. Once this is done we can then work with that individual/family together to meet their needs and provide the highest standard of person-centred care possible.

Boundaries

Boundaries have been discussed briefly in Chapter 3. It is important to understand that all relationships have boundaries, which assist us to establish the kind of relationship it is and to identify the rules and expectations within it. The relationship between the nurse and 'patient' is therapeutic and it is present because that particular individual has health and social care needs. These have a requirement to be addressed and the focus is on the health and welfare of the individual/family.

The relationship is not a friendship; rather it remains purely professional and it is important that the professional is aware of what might and might not be appropriate to disclose or discuss. For example it may be the case that the individual may ask a specific question in relation to the professional's private life or suggest the relationship develop further into a friendship or a relationship of a sexual nature. There needs to be an acknowledgement that this would not be appropriate or acceptable and conflicts with the NMC Code of Conduct (NMC 2008).

There is also a need to be aware of interdependence and the degree that each individual is dependent on the other. Building a rapport and a therapeutic relationship is important but it is possible for the 'patient' to become too dependent on the nurse. This can result in ethical issues and conflict and can be avoided by professionals working inter-professionally and as a team. Within the community this may be facilitated by different members of the nursing team sharing visits to that patient and family while still maintaining continuity of care.

The practitioner must be clear in relation to their role and the therapeutic relationship and adhere to the NMC Code of Conduct (NMC 2008), remaining accountable and maintaining clear boundaries.

Power

We all have power in some aspect of our lives (Haugaard 2002); the first step is for us to recognize where this power may lie. As nurses it may be perceived to be in the uniform we wear, the role or title we hold or the attitude and behaviour we display. This may be considered oppressive by patients within their own care setting and intrusive of their own privacy. We need to recognize when this might be the case and use 'power' to the benefit of the person involved to avoid this occurring within practice.

This concept is important to consider in the assessment process. In the context of community nursing individuals can easily feel 'oppressed' if we do not respect the fact that we are a guest who the 'patient' has invited into their home or care setting. A professional entering someone's home and exerting power to control that individual or particular situation may result in feelings of resentment, intimidation and anxiety. The visit may well be perceived as intrusive and affect the partnership working and 'therapuetic relationship'. Equally patients can feel overwhelmed and that they have no choice but to follow the professional's advice and therefore not participate fully in their care and decision making.

Reflection

How do you review your practice in relation to oppression and what might your identified developmental needs be which you may choose to include within your personal development plan?

You may have identified the following:

- not respecting the person as an individual;
- not utilizing effective communication and not listening to the individual, their 'story' and what is important to them;
- assuming how you may address them or using language which may be considered as condescending, for example 'love', 'sweet', 'darling', 'honey' or perhaps using their first name as opposed to 'Mrs Brown';
- forming preconceived ideas in relation to what the individual's health needs may be and becoming too over prescriptive in relation to referrals, service provision and how you feel the care should be managed;
- not respecting the patient or the carer for 'the expert' they may be in relation to their condition or circumstances.

Assessment

The National Health Service (NHS) and Community Care Act (DH 2008) was introduced to govern health and social care. The legislation set out how the NHS and local authorities should assess and provide for patients' health and social needs. The Act introduced an internal market which encouraged trusts to compete and provide health and social care and promoted the state as an enabler rather than a supplier of health and social care provision. Needs assessment is a key component of the community nurse's (district nurses – DN) role like many other primary care workers. DNs and social workers were identified as key professionals within the assessment of health and social needs. The process requires a skilled professional to complete a comprehensive and accurate assessment preferable jointly and in partnership if it is relating to both health and social needs.

The reasons for this will be discussed later in the chapter but an important part of this is to ascertain exactly what the health and social needs are so that they can be funded appropriately either by health or social care. For patients like Evie Brown (case scenario 1, Chapter 1) receiving care there may seem like an unclear divide between health and social needs and how these will be paid for. For professionals it is paramount that an understanding of funding and service provision is achieved if timely referrals, services and resources are to be utilized to their maximum potential.

Reflection

Consider the funding of health and social care. Once assessment needs have been identified a decision needs to be made as to whether each need should be met by health or social care. Remember health care is free at the point of delivery, however social care requires an individual financial assessment. Depending on the outcome of this financial assessment the 'patient' or 'service user' may or may not have to contribute to the funding of their social care. It may also mean that the individual could be eligible to pay for all their social care. However, if the health and social needs are complex the individual may meet the 'continuing care' eligibility criteria. 'Continuing care' means care provided over an extended period of time, to an individual aged 18 or over, to meet physical or mental health needs that have arisen as a result of disability, accident or illness. 'NHS continuing health care' means a package of continuing care that is arranged and funded solely by the NHS.

Case scenario 1 (Chapter 1) related to Evie Brown who had fallen and sustained a severe sprained left ankle with a small skin tear. A referral was made to the DN by the out of hours community nurses for further assessment in relation to the fall and also to dress the wound.

Assessment is complex and we must not be lulled into the misconception that it focuses primarily on physical need. Benner et al. (2009) discusses the continuum and journey from novice to expert that professionals move along developing on their experience and knowledge, perhaps never achieving complete expertise (see Figure 7.1). Benner clearly argues that practice without theory cannot produce fully skilled nurses; however, theory without practice has even less chance of success.

You as student nurses will make this same journey along the continuum developing from novice to expert although it may be argued that we never reach the 'expert' phase as we are lifelong learners. When applying Benner's concept to assessment you will identify with the novice and advanced beginner role at the beginning of your training. This is likely to result in you initially being more reliant on a model of nursing, the nursing process and documents such as *The Essence of Care* (DH 2010). You may find that you use these tools and documentation and 'tick the boxes' to ensure you have collated all the important and relevant information in relation to assessment and care planning.

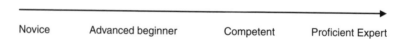

| Novice | Advanced beginner | Competent | Proficient Expert |

Figure 7.1 Benner's levels of nursing experience
Source: Benner (1984)

However, as the practitioner moves towards the end of the continuum to achieve expertise it can be observed that there is less dependence on these forms of documentation which originally may have been used as rigid tools within the assessment process. Instead they are used as guidelines and frameworks which underpin the assessment process as practitioners 'fine tune' their assessment and communication skills to discuss and identify needs in partnership with patients demonstrating the ability to elicit and prioritize needs incorporating the service user's perspective. It is at this stage where practitioners are able to have a conversation with the individual and/or family while completing the assessment, simultaneously gathering essential information and identifying in partnership what health and social needs may exist and how to coordinate care to manage these effectively.

Bradshaw (1972) discussed the identification of health need under four headings: normative need (as defined by professionals and experts); felt need (those people perceive for themselves); expressed need (when the felt need progresses to a demand); and comparative need (where one person's needs can be evaluated in relation to the provision of others). However, Cowley et al. (2000) reiterates that the concept of need remains subjective, individual, variable and changes. As professionals we may need to decipher and negotiate with the individuals whether it is truly a need or a want.

Most importantly practitioners must be aware of their own behaviour and responses so when individuals are met for the initial assessment professionals have not already identified normative needs and become ignorant of the individual's felt and expressed needs. This may be considered oppressive and an invasion of privacy and choice by that individual, resulting in disempowerment and putting the practitioner in conflict with the ethos of individualized and person-centred care.

Question

Considering assessment in relation to case scenario 1, what considerations would you make after receipt of the referral and prior to your visit to Mrs Brown?
   You may have listed some of the following:

- clarification of the referral details and initiate contact with the referee if appropriate and required;
- elicit information such as past medical history (PMH), previous notes, other professionals' involvement;
- contact Mrs Brown to introduce yourself, provide the rationale for your contact and gain consent to visit. Provide Mrs Brown with details of how she may contact you. You may find that because of Mrs Brown's forgetfulness you may need to consider gaining consent which would

enable her daughter Elizabeth to be present during your visit to support a holisitic approach to the assessment;

- ensure Mrs Brown is aware that she may wish to invite a friend/member of the family such as Elizabeth or significant other to be present at the meeting, perhaps to act in an advocacy or support role or to supplement information provided;
- Ensure you know the location, how to get there, parking arrangements (see Chapter 3) and have agreed a date for your visit and, in some cases, a specific time. It might be the case that Mrs Brown is not always at home and therefore essential you establish when you will be visiting to avoid wasted time and resources and ineffective communication.

 Reflection

Consider your lone working policy and ensure your team knows who you are visiting and when with an estimated time of return back to the community nursing base as well as access to both your and your line manager's contact details so either you or your manager may contact each other if needed.

Be aware that the information you obtain prior to the initial assessment visit should not influence your judgement in any way but aid the assessment process and enable you to engage Mrs Brown as quickly as possible. There are always advantages and disadvantages to accessing information about an individual prior to meeting them and you must ensure you have an awarenesss of how this may strengthen preconceived ideas, judgements and stereotyping. Bradshaw (1972) alludes to this concept when discussing normative need.

Bear in mind the contrast to an acute setting where multi-disciplinary teams (MDT) may meet together to discuss a patient's care. In the community setting the initial visit may be made in isolation by the community nurse; however, if required a joint meeting may be held in the individual's home with, for example, a social worker and a community nurse. This would be the preferred way of approaching joint assessment with the involvement and communication of other professionals involved. However, it does not generally imply that all the professionals would meet together in the patient's home. This may appear quite oppressive and inappropriate to an individual such as Mrs Brown and we must continue to remember that we are invited guests in individuals' homes.

If Mrs Brown's daughter, Elizabeth, is present during the visit it may be useful to consider accommodating some time for you to talk to Mrs Brown alone. This will enable her to have the opportunity to discuss anything she may not wish to talk about in front of her daughter.

Quite often relatives can approach you when you are leaving 'to have a quiet word' and provide further information. Be mindful that your duty of care is to your patient but it can be extremely valuable to listen to friends and family to gain further insight into family dynamics and ultimately a more holisitic assessment can be achieved.

The visit

On arrival wait to be invited into Mrs Brown's home and for her to direct you to where she would like you both to go. At this point you can introduce yourself, explain your role and establish why Mrs Brown thinks you are there. It also enables boundaries to be introduced, a relationship to be initiated and a rapport developed.

It is good to note at this point the environment and the context in which you are working. For example how long did it take Mrs Brown to open the door (you could ensure colleagues were aware of this). Are there stairs, unlevel surfaces or obstructions that would inhibit her mobilizing safely or that would pose a risk to this? Perhaps there are adaptations already in the home (such as the accommodation of washing and toilet facilities on the ground floor and the conversion of the dining room into a bedroom for Mrs Brown). Consider how Mrs Brown mobilizes and whether she currently uses any aids and how she uses these to mobilize. Don't forget to note Mrs Brown's appearance as both this and her behaviour may provide useful insight into her health and social circumstances.

Consider whether Mrs Brown may ask you to remove shoes for example, and also whether you can turn telecommunications such as mobile phones on silent.

Remember to discuss confidentiality as per the NMC code (2008) and consent for information to be shared with other professionals who may be involved on 'a need to know basis'.

Avoid using medical terms and jargon and ensure you speak slowly and clearly, periodically checking that Mrs Brown understands what you have said and that you repeat information to check you have understood what Mrs Brown has said. Consider impairments such as hearing and sight and whether Mrs Brown has her glasses or her hearing aid on and working.

Use your non-verbal communication and observational skills to identify if there are any issues in relation to effective communication such as those discussed above or how Mrs Brown and her daughter may be feeling with you as a stranger although a professional present in their home.

Ascertain how Mrs Brown would like you to address her – make no assumptions and consider your use of language. Avoid terms such as 'honey', 'love', 'sweetie', 'darling'. These may be considered condescending. Consider the use of touch and whether it would be appropriate at this juncture of the assessment – it might encroach on Mrs Brown's privacy and be considered too intimate so early on in the therapeutic relationship. Some people would never feel comfortable with the idea of touch and this is something you may need to establish as your relationship progresses.

Remember assessment is a continual process and therefore the assessment may not be completed on that initial visit. It may be appropriate for you to agree another time with Mrs Brown to return and continue the assessment process to engage partnership working and ownership by Mrs Brown of her own care. Furthermore this will facilitate the promotion of independence, self determination and empowerment.

 Question

What might you consider in relation to your verbal and non-verbal communication strategies during your visit to Mrs Brown?

You may have noted some of the following:

- Gestures such as smiling and nodding your head affirm to Mrs Brown that you are interested, willing to listen and engaged. Avoid looking at your watch as this may suggest you are in a rush and do not have time to listen.
- Your body position should be open, leaning forward without arms crossed to invite Mrs Brown to talk with you and demonstrate your interest. Creating barriers like having crossed arms or slouched in the chair/sofa may imply that you are not interested and cannot be bothered.
- Observe and acknowledge any non-verbal behaviours exhibited by Mrs Brown that may suggest she is uncomfortable or defensive about the current discussion or questions that are being asked.

 Discussion point

Consider whether you are asking closed or open questions.

Closed questions

These questions will often invite only yes or no or short factual answers with very little room to expand or elaborate. You will be required to probe further for more information. However, closed questions can enable you to get a specific answer or focus on something to gain clarification.

Open questions

These questions may start with 'how', 'what' or 'why' and enable Mrs Brown to think and reflect on her answer, provide opinions and feelings and have control over the conversation. This type of questioning will provide you with a longer answer, more information and will also demonstrate your interest in the conversation.

It may be that you need to periodically facilitate the conversation with phrases such as 'go on', 'umm' and 'please continue' to encourage Mrs Brown to proceed with her conversation.

Remember silence can be a useful tool to enable both yourself and Mrs Brown to reflect on what has been said and organize thoughts. People can feel uncomfortable with this and it can be a skill that you develop over time but don't think that just because no one is speaking that it is necessarily a bad thing.

Avoid using leading questions which may influence the response and only provide the answer you were looking for such as 'you don't go out without your wallking stick do you?' Mrs Brown could gauge from this you are hoping that she does not and therefore may not be truthful with her answer.

 Discussion point

Remember the earlier point that you should clarify what you think Mrs Brown has said and also repeat the information to avoid any misconceptions. It is also an opportunity for Mrs Brown to provide further explanation in relation to the information provided.

Don't forget to summarize and ensure you have collated the essential data and not just what you may feel is essential but what is also important and a priority for Mrs Brown. This also is a good way of informing Mrs Brown the visit is coming to an end and an opportunity for you to make another date to visit if required and check that Mrs Brown has nothing else she would like to tell you at that time.

Question

What information might you require for your initial visit? Make a list.
   You may have listed the following:

Ensure you have Mrs Brown's correct biographical information including her name, date of birth (address details you will have), marital status, nationality, religious preferences (and consider how this may affect diet, dress, day to day activities and health beliefs), who else may live at the address (such as her daughter, Elizabeth) and next of kin contact details (this may include work contact numbers), and her previous occupation as a headteacher.

Ask Mrs Brown what she believes to be her health problem. This may also include social problems such as personal care (remember Mrs Brown and her daughter pay for a formal carer who comes in daily to assist Mrs Brown with washing and dressing) and document her response accurately.

Discussion point

Discuss when the problem started and its progression and how this has affected her life and day to day ability to function. This will provide an opportunity for Mrs Brown to expand on her hobbies and interests such as her membership of the Castle Close's residents group. It should also assist in identifying what social support networks Mrs Brown has. As the case scenario states Mrs Brown and her daughter are supported by both neighbours and friends you may need to probe further to identify how they help.

From this discussion you should then be able to complete an assessment dependent on the module of nursing utilized within your own local area, identifying actual and potential needs for Mrs Brown. Initially as a novice you may find you are more reliant on this framework as a 'tick box' tool. It is likely you will be dependent on your mentor to guide you in identifying other information that would be essential to include and how to prioritize this in accordance with what Mrs Brown and her daughter have told you. However as you work along the novice to expert continuum you will develop and enhance your assessment skills. Eventually your assessment will develop and become a discussion with the nursing assessment model purely there as a framework for you to build your holistic assessment upon. You will have an increased ability and skill to observe your environmenal and contextual surroundings and elicit the information required while utilizing your verbal, non verbal and interpersonal skills to 'read between the lines' during the conversation.

Discussion point

It is useful at this point to find out how Mrs Brown feels about herself, her identity and how she may feel her role has changed within the community. Use this as an opportunity to identify any associated mental health issues.

Consider whether she feels safe at home and, if not, why not and when? This may not just be in relation to her recent history of falls and we should always remember that the professional's role is also to safeguard and observe those that are vulnerable. This issue is explored in Chapter 4. Do remember that you are obligated to report any type of abuse and should inform the patient that you would be required to do this. When we as professionals are aware of adults receiving care from family and friends we are responsible for assessing whether there are any issues of safeguarding that require addressing and must follow local policy in relation to this.

Reflection

Had you thought about Mrs Brown's daughter and what her needs may be?

Every informal carer has an automatic right to a carer's assessment and this choice must be offered to Elizabeth. If she consents to this offer, social services would provide this assessment which would identify with Elizabeth any actual or potential needs. This could include respite care or the use of voluntary organizations. It should be made clear that the assessment will identify need but cannot guarantee it will be met and this depends on local service provision and funding. Just as you noted Mrs Brown's appearance and behaviour, do the same with Elizabeth. Again this can provide you with a useful insight in relation to how she may be coping or managing with her mother's health and social needs.

Documentation

The NMC *Record Keeping: Guidance for Nurses and Midwives* (NMC 2009) which also makes reference to the *Data Protection Act* (1998) is clear that we must document our actions accurately and comprehensively to maintain our accountability. This ensures that evidence supports communications with patients and families, continuity of care and how clinical judgements and decisions are agreed. Effective documentation also helps to identify risks and early detection of communication issues, assists with the audit cycle and improving care, and demonstrates the provision of services that have been offered and referred to. If documentation is not completed there is absolutely no evidence of what has or has not been discussed, agreed or provided.

Assessment must be accurate and as comprehensive as possible. This will enable need to be identified effectively and enhance continuity of care between professionals and for Mrs Brown. It should also be completed in partnership with Mrs Brown and her daughter Elizabeth. An example of what a completed assessment might entail is given in Table 7.1. This shows a completed assessment with Mrs Brown using Roper et al.'s (1980) model of nursing identifying actual and potential health and social needs.

Question

What other risk assessments might you discuss with Mrs Brown and Elizabeth after completing this assessment?

You may have considered the following:

- falls risk assessment
- manual handling risk assessment
- pressure sore risk assessment
- nutritional screening risk assessment
- bowel assessment
- depression screening
- carer's assessment

Question

What referrals may you discuss with Mrs Brown and Elizabeth?

You may have considered the following:

- Referral to GP for recent memory loss. Request blood screen and medication review. (Consider urine dipstick for abnormalities.)
- Dependent on diagnosis consider possible referral to specialist in dementia care and support services/memory clinic/day services.
- Consider and discuss occupational therapist (OT) and physiotherapist referrals to assess mobility and daily functioning in respect for adaptations and provision of equipment. The aim to minimize risk of falls and maximize safety in the home.
- Consider and discuss social services referral with Mrs Brown and also carer's assessment for Elizabeth.
- Discuss service provision in voluntary sector to support Elizabeth and facilitate further respite.

Table 7.1 Completed assessment with Mrs Brown

Activity of living	Comments	Actual (A) or potential (P) problem
Maintaining a safe environment	At risk of falling. Two steps up to front door. Lives in terrace house with 18 stairs to upstairs level (narrow and steep) but adaptations recently made. Washing and toilet facilities are also now downstairs and dining room converted into bedroom. Downstairs there is a walk-in shower with shower chair and non slip mat. One rug in hallway. Her daughter Elizabeth (only child) lives in house and sleeps upstairs. Centrally heated. Downstairs all on one level. Elizabeth prompts her mother to take her oral medications which are in a nomad tray with written instructions as a reminder. The last medication review was completed seven months ago by the GP and the nomad is collected from the pharmacist on a weekly basis.	A
Communication	Over the past nine months Mrs Brown has become increasingly forgetful from not remembering names to forgetting where she has put things, who people are and where she has been. Mrs Brown wears glasses for both distance and near sight and a hearing aid in her left ear. If you sit in front of Mrs Brown, maintain eye contact and speak slowly but clearly she will understand you. Mrs Brown needs reminding to check her hearing aid battery works as she forgets to do this at times. Mrs Brown has a computer and enjoys using the Internet but her failing memory impacts on her ability to remember what she has or has not done. She maintains some of her social networking via email. Generally Mrs Brown is a private person.	A
Breathing	Mrs Brown has no presenting difficulties with breathing. Her respirations are 19 on rest and 24 after exertion. Her pulse is 84 beats per minute and blood pressure 134/85. No history of respiratory or cardiac disease. Mrs Brown has never smoked.	Not at present

(Continued)

Table 7.1 (Continued)

Activity of living	Comments	Actual (A) or potential (P) problem
Eating and drinking	Mrs Brown has a small appetite and tends to snack three or four times during the day. She generally has a balanced nutritional intake and her daughter Elizabeth prepares an evening meal and some snacks during the day with a flask of tea and juice available. Mrs Brown requires prompting to eat her snacks and Elizabeth has to telephone and remind her if she is not there. Mrs Brown does not require assistance with eating and drinking only prompting and her favourite meal is fish pie and a cup of tea. On the weekend she likes a glass of wine with her Sunday roast. Mrs Brown wears dentures which Elizabeth cleans on a daily basis and soaks overnight. Without these Mrs Brown cannot chew on her food.	P
Elimination	Mrs Brown has access to toilet facilities downstairs and is able to get to these unsupervised but requires reminding to use the toilet but manages independently. She has a hand rail to assist her to get on and off the toilet. When Elizabeth isn't there and has to ring her mother to remind her to eat her snacks she also reminds her to use the toilet. At night Mrs Brown uses a commode by her bed to micturate (usually once). Mrs Brown is continent but is prone to constipation. Her normal elimination pattern for opening her bowels is every other day, usually in the morning. Elizabeth self administers Senna tablets if her mother does not maintain this pattern to avoid impaction and also encourages her mother to mobilize and drink fluids and modifies her diet with increased fruit and vegetables.	P
Washing and dressing	Elizabeth has a formal carer paid privately (Mrs Brown has previously declined offer of help via social services) who visits every morning usually around 9am to assist Mrs Brown with washing and dressing. Mrs Brown can do her own face, hands and front part of her body but requires help with the rest. The carer washes Mrs Brown's hair twice weekly and cuts her nails. The mobile hairdresser visits every fortnight and the chiropodist (from the local medical centre) completes a domiciliary visit once every month. Mrs Brown likes to wear make up every day and Elizabeth paints her mother's nails – her favourite colour is pink.	A

Activity	P/A	Notes
Controlling body temperature	P	Mrs Brown requires prompting to adjust bed linen and wear appropriate clothing dependent on where she is going and weather. Her carer assists with this in conjunction with Elizabeth. Her normal body temperature is just below 37 degrees. Mrs Brown does not like to feel too hot and gets agitated if she does.
Mobilization	A	Mrs Brown has got one stick but forgets to use this and also has said to Elizabeth that she does not want people to think she is old, disabled or not able to participate in 'normal' community life. Mrs Brown wears slippers at home and 'Cosey' Velcro shoes when out. She has sustained from her recent fall a severe sprained left ankle with small skin tear.
Working and playing	A	Mrs Brown was a festival trustee for the local arts and music festival for many years and has a music prize set up in honour of her husband who was a local councillor. Mrs Brown feels very low that she has been unable to attend the Castlefields residents group due to her recent forgetfulness. Mrs Brown has one child, Elizabeth, a retired headteacher who is an active member of the gardening society, a voluntary guide at the museum and has a role within the Minster church community. Elizabeth has been living with her mother for the past three months. Support from friends and the employed carer have enabled Elizabeth to pursue her hobbies and interests. Mrs Brown is keen to access her church and the vicar visits once weekly.
Expressing sexuality	P	Also see notes under washing and dressing. Mrs Brown was widowed 15 years ago (married 60 years ago) and has close male friends (Bill is her closest friend and lives nearby) but no relationships of an intimate nature. She likes to get dressed up and attend social functions with her various clubs although the frequency of this has reduced with her recent memory loss.
Sleeping	P	Mrs Brown sleeps throughout the night and has a commode near her bed to reduce the risk of falls when she gets up to use the toilet to micturate (usually once). During the day Mrs Brown usually has a short sleep in the afternoon if at home.
Death and dying	A	There was not sufficient time to discuss this issue at length with Mrs Brown on the first visit but during the assessment her daughter mentioned that her mother had said on many occasions 'that if she knew she had dementia she would not want to go on' if she could not remember anything or had no recollection of events. Elizabeth became quite tearful at this stage and left the room. We chatted before I left and agreed on a further discussion and made another date to visit again. Mrs Brown did add when I was leaving that she will never leave 'unless in a box'.

The following is a discussion in relation to the assessment for the resident within case scenario 2. The principles of communication, interpersonal skills and professionalism remain the same as do the preliminary enquiries prior to your visit which require transferrable skills.

Essie and Marvin West have three children and live on the new housing estate in Chettlesbridge. Essie has recently been diagnosed with breast cancer and had a mastectomy several weeks ago. Essie has been warned that the cancer is aggressive and the prognosis is not good as the tumour has spread. She is to undergo chemotherapy.

Essie's mother lives in Trinidad and is too ill to travel. Her father died several years ago and her two sisters live in America. Marvin's family live in London but the relationship is strained. He does not get on with his mother.

The children are aware that Essie has cancer but they do not know that the prognosis is poor. The middle child is having nightmares and is becoming very anxious at being separated from her mother. She is 7 years old.

 Question

What considerations would you make after receipt of the referral and prior to your visit to Mrs West?

You may have considered the following:

- clarify the referral details and initiate contact with the referee if appropriate and required;
- elicit information such as past medical history (PMH), previous notes, other professionals' involvement such as the oncology team, palliative care nurses, GP, family liaison professional;
- contact Mrs West to introduce yourself, provide the rationale for your contact and gain consent to visit. Provide Mrs West with details of how she may contact you. You may need to ascertain whether Mrs West requires or wishes Mr West to be present during your initial meeting;
- ensure you know the location, how to get there, parking arrangements and have agreed a date for your visit and in some cases a specific time;
- remember your lone working policy.

Question

What information may you require for your initial visit to Essie and Marvin?
  You may have considered the following:

- Ensure you have Mrs West's (Essie) correct biographical information such as her name, date of birth (you will have address details); marital status, nationality, religious preferences (and consider how this may affect diet, dress, day to day activities and health beliefs); who else may live at the address (such as her husband/three children) and next of kin contact details (this may include work contact numbers).
- Remember at this point it is essential to listen to Essie and Marvin and facilitate an opportunity for them to talk to you about their thoughts and feelings at this present time, what their priorities are and also to express any particular issues of concern.
- It is also essential that you elaborate on your role and the part you will play in working with them to manage care as effectively as possible.

Question

What could your role involve as a community nurse?
  You may have considered the following:

- navigator and coordinator of care and the ability to signpost to other services/professionals and ensure appropriate, comprehensive, timely referrals made with consent;
- facilitating effective collaborative and inter-professional working;
- enabling continuity and seamless delivery of care;
- working in partnership with Mr and Mrs West to assess (both have given permission to address them by their Christian first name), identify needs and facilitate appropriate service provision with an awareness and acknowledgement of any cultural needs;
- champion and advocate for Mrs West and family;
- to provide service to meet health needs;
- to act as information provider and educationalist in relation to Mrs West and her family.

People approaching end of life require care in a variety of settings. An essential part of Essie's assessment would involve a discussion ascertaining what her wishes and preferences would be as she approached the end of her life. There is no right time to introduce this topic as it is so individualized and may be introduced by Essie, Marvin, other family, friends or by the professional. However it is important that Essie's preferred priorities for care (PPC) are identified as soon as possible in order for planning to occur. This will need to be continually reviewed and documented as Essie's wishes, preferences and priorities may change.

DH (1990) states that most people will spend the large majority of their last year of life within the community and may require a variety of services from both health and social care to enable them to continue to live and die at home if this is their choice. *The Gold Standards Framework* (GSF) enables primary and secondary care to work together to enable continuity of care, teamwork, advance life planning, symptom control and support for the patient, carer and staff.

The GSF has an indicator set for the *Quality Outcomes Framework* (QOF) within primary care and attracts points for GPs. Each GP practice establishes a register for all of those requiring end of life care and this ongoing care is reviewed at set multi-disciplinary meetings. The outcome is intended to provide more focused patient care and enhance care provided out of hours.

The Audit Commission study (1999) demonstrated that caring for people approaching end of life represents a large proportion of community nurses work which encompassed 40 per cent of a district nurse's time but only 8 per cent of their caseload.

 Question

Can you think of some different settings where people approaching end of life may require care?
You may have listed the following:

- acute hospitals;
- the community (in a person's home);
- care homes and sheltered and extra care housing;
- hospice;
- community hospitals;
- ambulance services;
- prisons and secure hospitals;
- hostels for the homeless.

Question

What services might be required to facilitate Essie dying at home?
  Consider the following:

- primary care;
- continuing care;
- private, independent and voluntary services;
- palliative care services;
- family liaison services;
- health visitor/counsellor/school nurse;
- counselling;
- pharmacist;
- out of hours.

Question

After reading the case scenario above can you suggest what other social issues
may be identified?
  Some suggestions are listed below.

Essie's mother lives in Trinidad and is too ill to travel. Her father died several
years ago and her two sisters live in America. How will Essie wish to manage this
situation and does she wish her family to be aware of the recent change in her
health status and that she is terminally ill? The issue of who would facilitate this
and how may need to be addressed.

Marvin's family live in London but the relationship is strained and he does not
get on with his mother. Will Essie want to inform Marvin's mother?

The present circumstances relating to the family dynamics may mean that
Essie does not have an extended family to rely on for support or to assist her,
Marvin and the chidren as her condition deteriorates. Independent and voluntary
organizations would need to be considered as with any individual or family should
Essie wish to have increased support or perhaps respite. 'It should be recognised
that not all carers are family members and not all family members are carers' (DH
2008).

Essie's children are currently unaware of their mother's prognosis. The middle child who is 7 years old is experiencing nightmares and anxiety at being separated from her mother. Useful resources such as the school nurse, health visitor and counsellor may also be utilized to support the family. The palliative care team may also be considered to discuss with Essie and Marvin how they wish to manage this situation. This can be facilitated by working with the family to develop a supportive environment where the children can be included and aware of the situation in a managed and coordinated way. This would enable relationships between all to be strengthened through involvement of a family liaison professional and provide an opportunity together and separately for those involved to express their own thoughts and feelings. It may also enable Essie to prepare and plan in a timely manner for her own death and memories for her family.

It is worth noting at this point that although this might be considered best practice it is Essie's choice whether she chooses to disclose to her children her prognosis and in our endeavour as professionals 'to act in the patient's best interests' we must also acknowledge people's rights, choice and autonomy although this may result in ethical challenges within practice.

Care after Essie's death and bereavement support for the family would need to be readily available and offered to all. This is particularly important for children coping with the death of someone important in their lives. As the End of Life strategy states, 'the specific needs of bereaved children and adolescents should be recognised and information and support given in a way that is sensitive to their maturity and level of understanding' (DH 1990).

Table 7.2 shows a completed assessment with Essie using Roper et al.'s (1980) model of nursing identifying actual and potential needs for Essie.

 Question

What other risk assessments might you discuss with Essie and Marvin after completion of this assessment?
You may have considered the following:

- pressure ulcer risk assessment;
- nutritional risk assessment – currently managed by community dietician;
- falls risk assessment;
- manual handling risk assessment;
- bowel assessment;
- carer's assessment.

Table 7.2 Completed assessment with Essie

Activity of living	Comments	Actual (A) or potential (P) problem
Maintaining a safe environment	Essie lives in a two bedroomed house with stairs but has a toilet and bathroom on both levels. She is currently struggling to get up and down the stairs and often has to do this by shuffling on her bottom under the supervision of Marvin. We have discussed the possibility of a physiotherapist and occupational therapist referral to assess and suggest possible alternatives that will promote safety and minimize risk of falls.	A
	At risk of increased infection risk as Essie is likely to develop a suppressed immune system due to chemotherapy (neutropenia). Essie may be at risk of altered sensation such as tingling or numbness, pins and needles in her feet and hands (peripheral neuropathy). Essie may experience a balance difficulty as a possible side effect of chemotherapy.	
Communication	Essie is able to communicate verbally and express herself and has no problems in relation to sight or hearing. However she is aware as her condition deteriorates that the ability to express her own needs may be affected hence her desire to participate in advanced life planning and preferred priorities of care. Some chemotherapy can affect hearing and Essie may experience ringing in her ears (tinnitus), or not hear high pitched sounds well.	P
	Essie has said her children are unaware of her diagnosis but she does not know how to tell them. We have discussed this at some length and Essie was receptive to the suggestion of a family liaison professional to facilitate and provide support. Essie is also concerned Marvin has no one to talk to and Marvin agrees he would benefit from professional counselling and support from the primary care team.	
	Contact details for the Macmillan and Cancer backup websites and support networks have been provided and also for the community nurses and out of hours service.	

(Continued)

Table 7.2 (Continued)

Activity of living	Comments	Actual (A) or potential (P) problem
Breathing	Due to forthcoming chemotherapy Essie may be at risk of low haemoglobin, experience tiredness, lethargy, dizziness, aching muscles and joints and perhaps shortness of breath. Essie may be at greater risk of blood clots. At present although tired and lethargic she is experiencing no other symptoms.	A
Eating and drinking	Essie's appetite has decreased and she has been prescribed nutritional supplements by the community dietician and GP and eats small snacks throughout the day. She is currently seen once a fortnight by the dietician. However Essie is also at risk of nausea and vomiting, altered taste and mouth ulcers as a side effect of chemotherapy. At present Essie's mouth is pink, moist and free from infection and so is her tongue. She has all her own teeth which she brushes twice a day. Essie will require encouragement to ensure an adequate intake of fluids to maintain kidney function.	A
Elimination	Essie has no problems with her elimination patterns at present and is able to use the downstairs toilet. Usually she opens her bowels every other day but can be prone to constipation. Essie has been prescribed two sachets of Movicol daily as and when she requires relieving the constipation. A side effect of chemotherapy may be constipation or diarrhoea.	P
Washing and dressing	Essie's hair may become dry and brittle and the same in relation to her nails due to treatments and she may be at risk of hair loss. The thought of this worries Essie. She may find that her skin becomes very dry or slightly discoloured due to chemotherapy. At present Essie reports her skin integrity is intact. At present Essie is able to wash her face, hands and intimate parts of her body but requires assistance for the remainder and dressing. Marvin has been helping Essie up to present.	A
Controlling body temperature	Essie is aware of whether she is too hot or cold although this may alter if she experiences altered sensation in her feet and/or hands. Marvin assists her with adjusting clothing, bed linen, room temperature such as heating and opening of windows.	A

Mobilization	Essie does mobilize independently without aids but has a walking stick although she does not like to use this. Increasingly she is feeling very lethargic and acknowledges she may require more support to mobilize safely and minimize the risk of falls. Essie has enquired about the possibility of accessing a wheelchair so she could go out more often with Marvin and also a blue disability badge for their car.	A
Working and playing	Essie has found that activities such as shopping have stopped as she has been too tired. She enjoys watching the television, listening to the radio and reading a good thriller book. However she would like Marvin to have some time to himself and has enquired about support services to visit so he could have some time off.	A
Expressing sexuality	Essie has had a left mastectomy eight weeks ago and adjusted to altered body image. Essie has expressed her concerns in relation to intimacy and continuing a sexual relationship with Marvin primarily because of the mastectomy and declining libido. Essie would like to continue her normal personal routines for as long as possible and enjoys ensuring she is well presented and wearing make up.	A
Sleeping	Essie has interrupted sleep patterns which she feels is because she often sleeps throughout the day. She and Marvin sleep in separate beds at the moment so she does not disturb him when she awakes but finds her sleeping pattern manageable at present. As a possible side effect of the chemotherapy Essie may feel anxious, restless, tired or sleepy.	P
Death and dying	Planned chemotherapy. Essie and Marvin have openly discussed and asked questions re planning for future and advanced life planning. Have discussed priorities of care with Essie and she would like to remain and die at home as her condition deteriorates. However both Essie and Marvin have expressed some anxiety re expectations and how they will access support. The Liverpool care pathway has briefly been referred to and this will be revisited at a later date. Essie stated she found this 'reassuring'. Essie has agreed to referral to community palliative care team and follow up visit to discuss this further. Essie is a Baptist although she does not actively practise or attend church and would not wish for a church representative to visit in the future.	A

Question

What referrals may you discuss with Essie and Marvin?
   You may have considered the following:

- palliative care;
- gold Standards Framework;
- family liaison;
- social services;
- continuing care;
- independent, voluntary and private sector for support services including useful networking sites such as cancer backup/Macmillan;
- referral to allied health care professionals (physiotherapist and occupational therapist);
- manual handling support team for carers;
- counselling.

Chapter summary

After completing this chapter you should have recognized that assessment is a unique and complex experience and an ongoing process. It is dependent on the following:

- the effectiveness of your communication and interpersonal skills;
- the effectiveness of your assessment skills and insight into your working environment and context of care;
- your ability to facilitate individualized and person-centred care.
- Chapter 8 on care planning will expand further on the above assessments and the nursing process within the community context.

NMC Essential Skill Cluster (ESC)	ESC number
Care, Compassion and Communication	1, 2, 3, 4, 5, 6, 7, 8
Organizational Aspects of Care	9, 10, 11, 13, 14, 16, 17, 18
Nutrition and Fluid Management	27, 28, 30
Medicines Management	34, 35, 36, 39, 40

References

Audit Commission (1999) *First Assessments: A Review of District Nurse Services in England and Wales*. London: Audit Commission.

Benner, P. (1984) *From Novice to Expert: Excellence and Power in Clinical Nursing Practice*. Addison-Wesley. USA: Prentice-Hall.

Benner, P., Tanner, C. and Chesla, C. (2009) *Expertise in Nursing Practice*, 2nd edn. New York: Springer.

Bradshaw, J. (1972) The concept of human need. *New Society*, 30: 640–3.

Chapman, A. (2006) Johari Window. http://www.businessballs.com/johariwindowmodel.htm (accessed 16 June 2011).

Cowley, S., Bergen, A., Young, K. et al. (2000) A taxonomy of needs assessment, elicited from a multiple case study of community nurse education and practice. *Journal of Advanced Nursing*, 31(1): 126–34.

DH (Department of Health) (1990) *The National Health Service and Community Care Act*. London: HMSO.

DH (2008) *End of Life Care Strategy: Promoting High Quality Care for all Adults at the End of Life*. London: HMSO.

DH (2010) *Essence of Care*. London: The Stationery Office.

Goleman, D. (1996) *Emotional Intelligence: Why it Can Matter More than IQ*. London: Bloomsbury.

Haugaard, M. (ed.) (2002) *Power: A Reader*. Manchester: Manchester University Press.

McIntosh, J. (2006) The evidence base for individual and client assessment by community nurses. *Primary Health Care Research and Development*, 7(4): 299–308.

NMC (Nursing Midwifery Council) (2008) *The Code of Conduct: Standards of Conduct, Performance and Ethics for Nurses and Midwives*. London: NMC.

NMC (2009) *Record Keeping: Guidance for Nurses and Midwives*. London: NMC.

Rogers, C. (1951) *Client Centred Therapy*. London: Constable.

Roper, N., Logan, W.W. and Tierney, A.J. (1980) *The Elements of Nursing*. Edinburgh: Churchill Livingstone.

Useful websites

Gold Standards Framework (GSF) www.goldstandardsframework.nhs.uk.

Liverpool Care Pathway (LCP) www.lcp-mariecurie.org.uk

Marie Curie Delivering Choice Programme www.deliveringchoice.mariecurie.org.uk

NHS End of Life Care Programme www.endoflifecareforadults.nhs.uk

Preferred Priorities for Care (PPC) www.cancerlancashire.org.uk

8   Care planning

Introduction

This chapter reflects on the residents of the two case scenarios and completed assessments in Chapter 7 and asks you to consider the assessment process in relation to both scenarios within the community setting. This will once again help you reflect on community nursing and consider your own solutions within these given situations.

This chapter will consider:

- the role of care planning;
- the integration of the self care ethos within care planning;
- the skills and knowledge required to complete individualized and person-centred care plans within the community setting;
- documentation.

Learning outcomes

At the end of this chapter you should be able to:

- discuss the role of care planning and how care may be planned, implemented and evaluated in partnership with an individual and/or family to meet the identified health and social needs within the community setting;
- recognize the skills, theory and concepts that underpin individualized and person-centred care planning within the home setting;
- Consider ways of promoting self care when care planning.

Supporting People with Long Term Conditions: Commissioning Personalised Care Planning is a DH document released in 2009 which states the following:

Key elements of the care planning process:

- **puts the individual, their needs and choices that will support them to achieve optimal health and well-being** at the centre of the process;
- **focuses on goal setting and outcomes** that people want to achieve, including carers;
- **is planned, anticipatory and proactive** with **contingency** (or emergency) **planning** to manage crisis episodes better (for those with complex needs);

- **promotes choice and control** by putting the person at the centre of the process and facilitating better management of risk;
- **ensures that people**, especially those with more complex needs or those approaching the end of life, receive coordinated care packages, reducing fragmentation between services;
- **provides information** that is relevant, timely and accredited to support people with decision making and choices (e.g. supported by an **Information Prescription**);
- **provides support for self care** so that people can self care/self manage their condition(s) and prevent deterioration;
- **facilitates joined-up working** between different professions and agencies, especially between health and social care; and
- **results in an overarching, single care plan** that is owned by the person but can be accessed by those providing direct care/services or other relevant people as agreed by the individual, e.g. their carer(s). This may be a written or electronic document or may be something that is recorded in the person's notes. The important aspect of this is the care.

The document is clear that the care planning discussion has taken place with an emphasis on goal setting, equal partnership, and negotiation and shared decision making.

The Department of Health also published in February 2011 an 'at a glance' guide for health care professionals in relation to personalized care planning (DH 2011). It emphasizes that the aim of personalized care planning should be to empower individuals and promote independence and informed decision making in partnership with their carers. This is achieved by focusing on listening to individuals about what matters to them and exploring what support is required to meet identified needs. The key point to note is that it is recognized that there are many issues other than medical needs which affect a person's total health and well-being. Comprehensive and effective care planning enables management of care to be risk assessed, proactive and anticipatory and supporting self care promotes ownership and control by that person in relation to their health and social care needs.

Why do we care plan?

Care planning is a fundamental part of nursing and it is a requirement not only to be able to undertake a comprehensive and accurate nursing assessment but to be able to create and document a plan of nursing care where possible in partnership with patients, carers, family and friends within a framework of informed consent. The new standards for pre registration nurse education (NMC 2010) clearly state that 'all nurses must ascertain and respond to the physical, social and psychological needs of people, groups and communities. They must then plan, deliver and evaluate safe, competent, person-centred care in partnership with them, paying special attention to changing health needs during different life stages, including progressive illness and death, loss and bereavement.'

Care planning may be done by individualized care plans, core care plans and care pathways (these are standardized plans of care written for particular diseases and procedures). With the introduction of *Essence of Care* (DH 2010b) core care plans have become more familiar to nurses than individualized written care plans. This was a tool to promote patients' focused care and a culture of sharing and comparing practice. Specific fundamental aspects of care have had benchmarks (standards) assigned to them to drive forward best practice and provide an improved experience for individuals when receiving health and/or social care. However the ability to be able to create an individualized care plan should not be underestimated and is a skill that all nurses require. If you are able to competently produce an individualized care plan you should be able to demonstrate an understanding of the care that will be delivered and the rationale for this. Core care plans need to be compiled in the first place and there certainly is not a core care plan for every individual problem. Only a person with the required care planning skills will be able to do this and then adapt core care plans to suit individual needs.

'Personalised care planning is essentially about addressing an individual's full range of needs, taking into account their health, personal, family, social, economic, educational, ethnic and cultural background and circumstances' (DH 2009: 11). It is a holistic and cyclical process, incorporating risk management and proactive planning for anticipated circumstances, especially for those with complex health and social care needs. It should promote joined up working and coordinated provision of services to meet identified health and social needs. The result should be less duplication of information and a promotion of continuity of care for the individual.

It is paramount to remember that personalized care planning is a discussion and a negotiated process between the individual and the professionals and partnership working is pivotal to its success. It should be based on need/s of the individual and not on what services can be provided and should promote empowerment, self determination, choice and independence with the individual as central. People should be encouraged to participate in decision making and risks should be managed accordingly along with the facilitation of the concept of self care.

The nursing process (Yura and Walsh 1988) was introduced as a more structured approach in relation to delivering care. Assessment, planning, implementation and evaluation are the four elements of this process and it essentially underpins the decision-making process. As a student nurse you will be required to demonstrate your understanding of this process in tandem with a model of nursing. Both the model of nursing and the nursing process are used together in partnership with the patient to identify actual and potential needs, plan the care that will be delivered and how it will be implemented with a specific time frame for this to be reviewed and re-evaluated. The patient must be involved as much as possible if the care planned is to be person-centred and individualized and the goals are to be realistic and achievable.

Remember that it will not be possible to solve all problems and it may be that you need to consider small goals first and review and set new goals once these have been achieved. Goals may be used to alleviate problems or used proactively to prevent potential problems developing into actual problems. Whatever goals are agreed they should always be clear, mutually agreed when possible, realistic, measurable and possible to evaluate and may be short or long term.

When planning care for implementation it should be evidence based and you should be able to demonstrate your own accountability and rationale as to why specific interventions have been agreed.

Implementation of care needs to be tailored to the individual and the care setting acknowledging choice, values and belief systems of that person respecting dignity and privacy.

Promotion of self care and self management

As the population ages and lives longer the increased burden on the NHS is set to rise, there is therefore a need to proactively manage care needs including long-term conditions (DH 2006).

Self care is a term that includes people taking responsibility for themselves every day to stay fit, maintain good physical and mental health well-being and action to prevent illness or accidents as well as effectively manage minor ailments and long-term conditions.

As accountable practitioners it is 'everybody's business' to ensure that appropriate information, health promotion and health education are provided. When necessary individuals should be signposted to the right service or referred appropriately and in a timely manner to ensure their identified need is met. On occasion it may be clear there is an 'unmet need'; we must take this opportunity to identify and report the issue according to local policy and consider whether there is a service requirement and why that might be. One opportunity to address this issue is to suggest, discuss and incorporate this within the assessment and care planning process.

 Question

In what ways might you promote and embed self care within clincial practice? You might have considered the following:

- Educate and inform individuals about where might be the most appropriate place, person and service to obtain information, education or assistance to manage minor ailments, minor injuries and major injuries. Explain what services provide and why.
- Educate individuals to understand their condition/s and associated risk factors and promote proactive healthy lifestyle choices.

- Promote the understanding of treatment options and encourage individuals to actively participate in decision making about the management of their care to promote choice, independence and empowerment.
- Educate and ensure individuals understand what their medications are for, actual and potential side effects, when and how to take them.
- Promote people to take responsibility when appropriate in relation to medication review and the rationale for this.
- Encourage individuals to be proactive in relation to their medications and ensure they acquire repeat prescriptions and replacement medications in a timely manner to reduce the risk of an emergency situation.
- Engage individuals and where consent is obtained significant others within the care planning process in partnership to promote joint decision making and concordance.
- Educate individuals and where consent is obtained significant others in recognizing exacerbations or deterioration of their particular condition and what planned action to take and who to contact.
- Support and advise individuals and where consent is obtained significant others to manage the impact of the condition/s on their particular lifestyle. This should include emotional, psychological, spiritual, physical and social perspectives.
- Support individuals to build confidence to contact and use services including voluntary and the independent sector to enhance their health and social outcomes and quality of life.
- The use of assistive technology to manage risk and support people to remain at home within the community.

The following two reflection activities are self directed and you are required to complete two care plans in relation to the residents from Chettlesbridge in case scenarios 1 and 2 (refer back to Chapter 1 for the case scenarios). Answers for both can be found in the Appendix (p. 185).

 Reflection

With reference to case scenario 1 and the example assessment completed in Chapter 7 please complete the following care plan underpinned by both the module of nursing assessment and the nursing process, addressing both the identified actual and potential needs of Mrs Brown. Be mindful that this would need to be completed in partnership with Mrs Brown. Her consent would need to be obtained in relation to this process and sharing of information and also if her daughter Elizabeth was going to be involved. Promotion of independence, self empowerment and informed decision making should be fundamental aspects of this process. Mrs Brown is happy to be addressed either as 'Mrs Brown or Evie' and her daugher as 'Elizabeth'.

Problem and actual (A) or potential (P)	Goal/ objective	Implementation (interventions planned)	Evaluation	Review date

 ## Reflection

With reference to case scenario 2 and the example assessment completed in Chapter 7, please complete the following care plan underpinned by both the module of nursing assessment and the nursing process, addressing both the identified actual and potential needs of Mrs West. Remember that consent is still required to share any information or make any referrals from Mrs West. Promotion of independence, self empowerment and informed decision making should be fundamental aspects of this process. Mrs West has expressed she would like to be known as 'Essie' and Mr West as 'Marvin'.

Problem and actual (A) or potential (P)	Goal/ objective	Implementation (interventions planned)	Evaluation	Review date

Reflection

Consider using this care planning template to guide you when documenting the care planning process in practice.

Provision of care

 Question

How are services purchased to meet population need within primary care and how is this going to change with the introduction of the White Paper *Equity and Excellence: Liberating the NHS* (DH 2010a)?

At present primary care trusts (PCTs) hold 80 per cent of the budgets and while primary care services such as GPs identify the services that will meet the needs of their local geographical populations PCTs secure the contracts and provide all the administration and management of these which is overseen by the strategic health authority (SHA).

However with the introduction of the White Paper *Equity and Excellence*, both SHAs and PCTs are to be abolished and instead Clinical Commission Groups will be introduced, which will be regulated by Monitor (this currently regulates foundation trusts).

Clinical Commission Groups will be responsible for commissioning (buying) services to meet the needs of their local populations. GPs are considered 'the gateway' to all services for patients and together with other professionals within primary care, voluntary and independent sectors it would appear to be the most appropriate way of commissioning services to meet need, maintain patient continuity throughout their individual 'journey' and ensure choice. Financial consequences will depend on the quality of service delivered and continue to be linked to the quality outcomes framework (QOF) (a tool used to measure health outcomes) and whether patient health outcomes continue to improve. It will remain extremely competitive as organizations such as the NHS, independent, private and voluntary sector tender their contracts to commissioners for procurement.

 Reflection

Use the link below to read the White Paper. *Equity and Excellence: Liberating the NHS* (DH 2010a). Use the questions below to facilitate further analysis of this paper.

http://www.dh.gov.uk/en/Publicationsandstatistics/Publications/Publications
PolicyAndGuidance/DH_117353

- Do you consider the transition of commissioning to GP consortia would be perceived as a positive move within the NHS?
- What is the relevance of commissioning to individualized care planning?
- How will GP consortia commissioning impact on patient care?
- How will GP consortia commissioning influence practice and relationships between primary and secondary care?
- How confident are you in the regulators such as Monitor and the Care Quality Commission?
- Will GP consortia have the skills, staffing and knowledge base to deliver commissioning – who might they use to support them?
- How do you think health inequalities will be affected by the intrduction of GP consortia commissioning?

Chapter summary

This chapter has introduced some key issues in relation to care planning within community settings:

- Care planning is an individualized and person-centred process that is cyclical and requires a therapeutic relationship.
- Care planning requires completion with the individual and significant others (with consent) and is a holistic process which identified actual and potential problems acknowledging the surrounding care context.
- Care planning must acknowledge and integrate informed decision making and lifestyle choices but promote a culture of self care.
- This is a process aligned with assessment that is a fundamental part of community nursing and a required skill for all pre-registration nursing students.

NMC Essential Skill Cluster (ESC)	ESC number
Care, Compassion and Communication	1, 2, 3, 4, 5, 6, 7, 8
Organizational Aspects of Care	9, 10, 13, 16
Nutrition and Fluid Management	27, 28, 30
Medicines Management	34, 35, 36, 39, 40

References

DH (Department of Health) (2006) *Supporting People with Long term Conditions to Self Care – A Guide to Developing Local Strategies and Good Practice*. London: Central Office of Information.

DH (2009) *Supporting People with Long Term Conditions: Commissioning Personalised Care Planning*. London: DH.

DH (2010a) *Equity and Excellence: Liberating the NHS*. Norwich: The Stationery Office. http://www.dh.gov.uk/prod_consum_dh/groups/dh_digitalassets/@dh/@en/@ps/documents/digitalasset/dh_117794.pdf (accessed 24 August 2011).

DH (2010b) *Essence of Care*. Norwich: The Stationery Office.

DH (2011) *Personalised Care Planning: An 'At a Glance' Guide for Health Care Professionals*. http://www.dh.gov.uk/dr_consum_dh/groups/dh_digitalassets/documents/digitalasset/dh_124048.pdf (accessed 7 November 2011).

NMC (Nursing Midwifery Council) (2010) *The New Standards for Pre Registration Nurse Education*. Norwich: The Stationery Office.

Yura, H. and Walsh, M. (1988) *The Nursing Process*, 5th edn. Norwalk, CT: Appleton and Lange.

9 The impact of nursing care

Introduction

This chapter aims to explore the impact of nursing interventions on health. Quality of care will be explored specifically related to the health and specific nursing interventions required by the residents of Chettlesbridge. It will consider the way in which community nurses can contribute to the continuous improvement of health care provided and the experiences of patients. The notion of nursing outcomes and the specific needs of some of the residents of Chettlesbridge have been discussed in previous chapters. The outcomes of nursing care and the ways in which nurses can be involved in the continuous improvement of health will be explored through further consideration of the residents of Chettlesbridge.

This chapter covers:

- health outcomes;
- measuring the effectiveness of nursing intervention;
- improving the quality of care for improved health outcomes;
- evidence-based practice.

Learning outcomes

At the end of this chapter you should be able to:

- explain the issues related to providing quality care to improve health outcomes;
- recognize the skills and knowledge required to ensure high quality outcomes for patients;
- identify the frameworks that exist to support nurses and other health care professionals to reach and maintain standards that ensure high quality outcomes for patients.

The themes raised in this chapter should be read within the context of the Nursing and Midwifery Council (NMC) Code of Conduct for Nurses and Midwives (NMC 2008). In relation to high quality health outcomes section 41 is particularly relevant: 'You must partake in appropriate learning and practice activities that maintain and develop your competence and performance.'

High standards of care lead to improved health outcomes for the patients in your care. By continually updating knowledge and skills, patient care is delivered to the best possible standard. The requirements for continuous professional development will be discussed further in Chapter 11.

Health outcomes

The improvement of population health has been high on the agenda of successive governments with publications and policy since the late 1990s focused on improving health. Clear objectives are set out in recent policy documents (Department of Health (DH) 2010a; 2010c) to ensure health improvements continue to be achieved. Quality initiatives with associated outcome measures have been identified within a framework of accountability that further ensures the performance of the NHS. It could be argued that the main outcomes of NHS care are:

- to improve the health of individuals and the population;
- to reduce the risks associated with ill health;
- to reduce the level of ill health by prevention and treatment;
- to reduce the number of premature deaths.

Health outcomes have been defined by the World Health Organization (WHO) (1998: 10) as: 'A change in the health status of an individual, group or population which is attributable to a planned intervention or series of interventions, regardless of whether such an intervention was intended to change health status'. This definition can be used to consider all aspects of health, including physical, mental and social health. This chapter will focus on the individual, while acknowledging the needs of groups and populations where appropriate. A change in health status is understood to be a positive change. The unintentional outcome of health intervention referred to in the definition above is an interesting concept and worthy of some exploration.

It could perhaps be assumed that all outcomes of a health or nursing intervention would be intentional; however the WHO definition above suggests that some are not. In Chapter 2 you were provided with a definition of health from the WHO and you have been introduced to the determinants of health. So you are familiar with the concept that being 'healthy' includes aspects of physical, mental and social well-being.

Consider some of the residents of Chettlesbridge:

- *Mrs Brown is very private and as such has employed a private carer to help with her personal care. The recent fall suffered by Mrs Brown has prompted a visit by the district nursing service. The referral suggested that the nursing intervention required was to re-dress a small ankle wound, sustained during the fall.*
- *Mary and her family live in a deprived area and have frequent visits from the community matron who monitors Eileen's respiratory condition.*
- *Larry and Michel are frequent visitors to the practice nurse who has been monitoring Larry's coronary heart disease and Michael's diabetes.*

Questions

Consider the residents' needs and the nursing intervention they are receiving. First, identify the intentional outcomes of the nursing interventions for the residents. You may have already identified some in Chapter 7 – did you consider the following?

- For Mrs Brown the intended outcome of nursing care could be seen as healing her wound and prevent further deterioration.
- The intention of the nursing care provided for Eileen is to help her manage her condition to prevent exacerbation and possible hospital admission.
- For Larry and Michel, again, the intended outcomes of nursing intervention might be to help them manage their long-term conditions and prevent them worsening.

As well as the above, what unintentional health outcomes could you identify that may arise from your initial involvement in the family?

As well as treating and maintaining physical health, you might have considered that social, environmental and mental health could be improved by the identification of issues such as:

- social isolation
- stress
- risk to safety
- need for health promotion/education
- maintaining independence.

Improvement in health has been identified as the desired outcome of any health-related intervention. It could be argued that good health outcomes are dependent on the quality of that intervention.

Quality of care

Quality care has been defined by many theorists; Martin et al. (2010), for example, provide an easy to digest chapter in their book *Managing in Health and Social Care*. A simple definition of quality care is provided by Gopee and Galloway (2009) who say quality is 'care delivery that meets a certain standard of excellence that is acceptable to both staff and patients' (Gopee and Galloway 2009: 86).

This definition will serve as a useful point to begin a discussion here. The definition includes some elements that require further scrutiny. Some questions arise from this definition such as:

- Whose standards are the best?
- Who defines excellence?

- What is acceptable to me or to you?
- Do both staff and patients agree?

This chapter does not intend to answer these questions or to provide a definition of quality for you to use. It does however intend to be a point of reference for you to begin to consider the issues to ensure your practice is based on accepted evidence that ensures high-quality outcomes for patients.

 Discussion point

Talk with your colleagues/mentor.
What could the consequences of poor quality care be?
What are the benefits of high quality care?
Did you discuss any of the following?
Poor quality:

- low patient satisfaction;
- low workforce morale;
- low 'productivity' and patient care;
- greater wastage of resources;
- higher costs.

High quality:

- higher patient satisfaction;
- better efficiency;
- increased morale of workforce;
- less waste.

Providing high quality care is required by law, the *Health Act 1999* section 18 – Duty of Quality – states: 'it is the duty of each Health Authority, Primary Care Trust and NHS trust to put and keep in place arrangements for the purpose of monitoring and improving the quality of health care which it provides to individuals.'

The NHS Constitution (DH 2010b) states two rights for patients associated with quality of care and environment:

1. 'You have the right to be treated with a professional standard of care, by appropriately qualified and experienced staff, in a properly approved or registered organisation that meets required levels of safety and quality';
2. 'You have the right to expect NHS organisations to monitor, and make efforts to improve, the quality of health care they commission or provide'.

(DH 2010b: 9)

The NHS Constitution (DH 2010b) also commits NHS providers:

1. 'to ensure that services are provided in a clean and safe environment that is fit for purpose, based on best practice (pledge)';
2. 'to continuous improvement in the quality of services you receive, identifying and sharing best practice in quality of care and treatments (pledge)'.

(DH 2010b: 9)

In short, patients have a right to high quality care and NHS organizations an obligation to provide or to ensure those organizations that are providing health care on their behalf are providing high quality care.

All elements of the care you provide to patients should be quality assured. Total quality management (TQM) is an approach to ensuring quality introduced by W. Edwards Deming into the Japanese manufacturing industry in the 1950s. It is based on the principle that a focus on customer satisfaction and continuous improvement will assure high quality products. While the NHS does not manufacture a product, it is committed to improvement and has recently adopted some of the principles and tools that support a TQM approach by:

- improvement is patient led;
- ensuring care is delivered by a motivated, highly trained workforce;
- ensuring a culture of continuous improvement is established;
- focusing on streamlining processes – processes are the problem, not people;
- getting things right the first time, improving quality and reducing costs;
- making decisions that are based on the best evidence.

Ensuring quality care for Mrs Brown

 Question

Look back at Chapter 8 where you were invited to complete a care plan for Mrs Brown. The care plan suggests a falls assessment is carried out; how might you ensure the effectiveness and quality of the falls assessment that you undertake?
You might have considered the following:

- Have you been trained to use the falls assessment tool?
- Is the tool a validated, reliable instrument? Will it provide accurate results?
- Is it clear what intervention should follow the assessment? Are these interventions available?

There is some evidence to suggest that not all falls assessment tools have the same levels of sensitivity and specificity (Chapman et al. 2011). Although this is an American study and has limitations, it does identify the importance of education in both the use of the tool and the subsequent interventions. An earlier study by Lovallo et al. (2009) also warns of the inaccuracy of falls assessment tools. They comment on the need for tools to be used in the same settings and used to assess the same populations as those they were tested on.

From the scenarios above, it is clear that the task of completing a falls assessment requires much preparation. The tools must be appropriate for the setting and the patient population they are used to assess. The nurse using the tool must be competent in its use. The results must be applied against a clear guideline. It could be argued that a falls assessment carried out by an inexperienced nurse using a tool that had been tested in a hospital setting for patients in their own homes would not provide an accurate assessment and therefore the possibility of a poor outcome for the patient is high.

Before using any assessment tool, ask yourself:

- Are you confident in the use of the tool?
- Are the processes clear for acting on the results?
- Is the tool endorsed by any other national guidance, e.g. NICE?

To minimize the risk of falls the care plan also states:

> To ensure Mrs Brown is provided with education, support and advice to promote safe mobilization. Provide practical information of how to minimize risk of falls around the home such as removal of rugs and a commode by the bed at night time.

 Question

How might you ensure that the education/information/support you provide for Mrs Brown is of high quality?

- You may have considered if there is any information readily available.
- Is it endorsed by a reputable organization, e.g. NICE, Age UK?
- Has it been prepared specifically for patients and carers?
- Is it in a format that your patient can read/hear?
- What equipment is available, is there a charge, how will it be maintained to ensure Mrs Brown's safety?

Evidence-based practice

Effective nursing requires the use of multifaceted skills and knowledge. Evidence-based practice has become part of the everyday vocabulary of nurses and other health care professionals. The need for evidence-based nursing practice is reinforced in the 2011 Government policy on the future of nursing and midwifery in England (DH 2011a).

Despite the evidence to suggest that patient outcomes are improved where evidence is underpinning practice, there is some concern about the way in which evidence is generally utilized in practice (Leufer and Cleary-Holdforth 2009). Aveyard and Sharp (2009) and Melnyk et al. (2010a) suggest that all available evidence should be used to underpin practice. They go on to say that this evidence should be a combination of sound clinical evidence, professional judgement and patient preference. The Royal College of Nursing (RCN) have developed a framework consisting of eight *Principles of Nursing Practice* (RCN 2010) that acknowledge these elements and support the delivery of quality nursing care that improves health outcomes and improves the patient experience. These principles according to Manley et al. (2011: 36) help nurses to 'demonstrate, measure and evaluate nursing practice' and 'assist patients in evaluating whether or not the care and treatment delivered by nurses meets their expectations'.

Using evidence to improve the quality of patient care

Consider the following scenario:

You have recently read an article about the benefits of a programme which provides education for people with long-term conditions. The programme aims to provide information for patients about combating fatigue, diet and exercise, managing pain and self-management. It can be delivered by trained health care assistants in the patient's own home. The article states that people who attend the programme require fewer visits to their GP. You think it may be a good idea for the residents of Chettlesbridge.

 Question

Ask yourself, would this type of programme reduce the number of GP visits for patients such as Larry and Michael and Eileen?

With an abundance of literature focused on the pursuit of evidence-based practice one might be excused for not quite knowing where to start answering the above question. Many frameworks exist.

Melnyk et al. (2010a) provide a step by step approach to using evidence-based practice, which consists of seven stages. These seven stages to evidence-based practice will be used to consider the question above.

0. Cultivate a spirit of inquiry

For evidence-based practice to flourish a development culture is needed. Creating a culture that embraces change is not easy. The NHS is a huge organization, a publically funded service that is continually responding to changes in the political, economic and social environment. It has to be responsive to new technological advances in medicines, Government policy and health crises such as swine flu, etc. The NHS is therefore subject to change due to influences that are unavoidable. However some changes can be made to the way care is delivered as a result of new knowledge or evidence. Melnyk et al. (2010a) suggest some questions that may help to promote 'a spirit of inquiry':

- *Who* can I seek out to assist me in enhancing my evidence-based practice knowledge and skills and serve as my evidence-based practice mentor?
- *Which* of my practices are currently evidence based and which don't have any evidence to support them?
- *When* is the best time to question my current clinical practices and with whom?
- *Where* can I find the best evidence to answer my clinical questions?

These questions may help to begin a discussion with colleagues about the evidence that supports practice. Reflection, journal clubs and clinical supervision can also provide vehicles for considering and questioning/discussing ideas for improvements to practice that are evidence based.

1. Ask clinical questions in a PICOT format

It is important that any potential changes to practice are appropriate. The PICOT format suggested by Melnyk et al. (2010b) provides the framework for clinical questions:

P – Patient population of interest
I – Intervention or area of interest
C – Comparison intervention or group
O – Outcome
T – Time

Now reconsider the original question in the PICOT format:

'For people in Chettlesbridge with long-term conditions (population) would attendance at a programme of education (intervention) compared to those who did not attend (comparison) reduce the number of GP visits (outcome) over a 6 month period (time)?

Using this format provides a question that contains key phrases that can be used in the second stage:

2. Search for the best evidence

Key search terms can easily be identified such as 'long-term conditions', 'programme of education', 'did not attend' and 'reduce GP visits'.

3. Critically appraise the evidence

Critical appraisal can be described as the systematic examination of research to confirm it is valid, reliable and trustworthy before using it to inform decisions about clinical practice. A concise guide *What is Critical Appraisal?* is provided by Burls (2009) and gives the novice a good introduction to what to consider in the pursuit of 'good evidence'. The Critical Appraisal Skills Programme (CASP 2010) provides checklists for all types of research papers and suggest three questions that can be applied to all research papers in the elimination of unhelpful publications. If the answer is 'yes' to the following questions, the paper may be worthy of a closer look:

- Is the study valid?
- What are the results? Are they clinically important?
- Are the results applicable to my needs?

4. Integrate the evidence with clinical expertise and patient preferences and values

As stated above research evidence is only part of what constitutes a good evidence base for practice. Consider what experience you and your colleagues may have had in this practice area. What is known about the patient's preferences for this type of intervention? Would patients be willing to participate?

If the evidence suggests the article was accurate in its statement of the benefits of the programme, implementation may be considered. The use of SMART objectives could be considered as a framework for setting objectives for the implementation of the project:

Specific: the programme will be available for participants in 12 months.

Measurable: a project plan should guide the implementation process. A timeline could be developed mapping each stage of the process to ensure the programme starts on time.

Achievable: ensure that all resources to manage the programme have been accounted for, including the staff.

Realistic: ensure a contingency plan is in place and that timescales have been carefully planned.

Timely: the programme is scheduled to begin during a time of low intensity work.

5. Evaluate the outcomes of the practice decisions or changes based on evidence

For any change to practice, evaluation is essential. Clear measurable outcomes should be stated. Both quantitative and qualitative data should be gathered. Measurable outcomes could include the following:

- How many patients were referred to the programme?
- How many patients started and completed the programme?
- How often did the patient visit the GP prior to the start over a 12 month period?
- How many visits to the GP were made in the 12 months following the programme?
- A questionnaire could be developed for patients to express their view and experience of the programme.

6. Disseminate evidence-based practice results

Sharing experiences with colleagues is important. This can be local or national. Nurses should be proud of their successes so share your work with others through journal articles, local media channels, professional organizations, etc. You might consider setting up a community of practice or a journal club in your workplace.

 Reflection

Consider your place of work:

- Is innovation encouraged?
- Do colleagues question practice?
- Is there opportunity for clinical supervision/discussion about practice development/improvement?
- Is practice ritualistic or evidence based?

If the answer to these questions is 'no' perhaps you could consider asking 'why?' Chapter 11 considers the attributes of leaders. Good clinical leadership is important in the development of a team in which innovative practice will flourish.

Effectiveness of nursing interventions

In previous chapters you have considered the interventions that are required for the residents and families of Chettlesbridge. It is apparent that nursing care must meet the needs of patients effectively.

Once health outcomes have been identified and interventions implemented there is a need for those interventions to be evaluated. Evaluation has been identified as the fourth element of the nursing process previously. Evaluation is a continuous process that helps nurses to consider the effectiveness of their interventions.

The outcomes of nursing interventions were first recorded by Florence Nightingale in 1854 (Nightingale 1854). The evidence presented by Florence Nightingale was in the form of statistical data that demonstrated the reduction in hospital deaths when nursing interventions were performed. Measurement of the effectiveness of nursing intervention requires specific outcomes to be identified and evaluated.

As part of its *Transforming Community Services* the DH (2011b) issued indicators for quality improvement for community services. The 43 quality indicators include measurable outcomes that can be used to identify where improvement is needed. The same measures can then be utilized following changes to care delivery and provide evidence for where improvements have been made.

Individual interventions can be evaluated by means of validated assessment measurement tools for interventions such as wound care, nutritional status, pressure sore risk, rehabilitation and treatment of depression. The RCN *Principles of Nursing Practice* (RCN 2010) include example measures for each principle; these could be incorporated and/or used alongside other evaluative tools. All outcome measures should be considered a way of improving quality of care. They can be used to inform the focus of local audit and patient surveys.

Clinical audit

Clinical audit has been defined by the Healthcare Quality Improvement Partnership (HCQIP) (2009) as: 'a quality improvement process that seeks to improve patient care and outcomes through systematic review of care and the implementation of change'. This definition is also endorsed by the National Institute for Health and Clinical Excellence (NICE). *The NHS Constitution* as discussed earlier refers to continual improvement and indeed one of the fundamental principles of TQM is that a culture of continual improvement is essential for quality.

The benefits of clinical audit have been described by the HCQIP (2009) as:

- promoting and enabling best practice;
- improving patient experience and outcomes;
- providing evidence that demonstrates where services are clinically and cost effective;
- providing opportunities for training and education;
- enabling better use of resources, and therefore, increasing efficiencies;
- improving communications and liaisons between clinicians, managers, patients and service users and organizations.

Clinical audit is often depicted as a cycle, demonstrating its continuous nature. There are many different representations of the audit cycle, one of which can be as in Figure 9.1. Each element of the cycle should be considered in sequence. Topics for audit could be considered for a variety of reasons including:

- the issue of new clinical guidelines, either national or local;
- poor patient outcomes from a specific intervention, specific clinical speciality;
- high cost interventions;
- a complaint or clinical incident.

Clinical audit of wound care in Chettlesbridge

Consider the following scenario.

Elizabeth Brown has called the nursing office today and has raised a concern about the way in which her mother Mrs Brown's leg wound is being carried out. She states that the wound has not been reviewed by a qualified nurse for six days. Her mother is complaining that her ankle is painful and 'smelly'. The community support worker Susan has told Miss

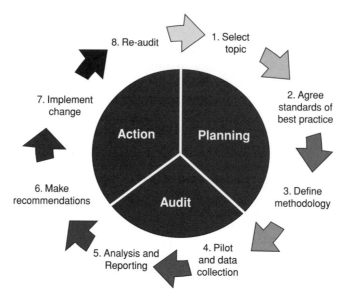

Figure 9.1 Clinical audit cycle
Source: Reproduced with kind permission from East Kent NHS Clinical Audit Service

Brown she thinks the wound may be infected. You review the wound and find that it is infected and that it has taken much longer to heal than anticipated. On further review of the caseload you discover that this is the fifth wound that has become infected in the past month.

You decide to conduct an audit to establish the effectiveness of wound care within the team to establish whether 'best practice is being practised'.

 Question

How might you go about establishing the effectiveness of wound care within the nursing team in Chettlesbridge?

Did you answer 'clinical audit'? This would be an effective way to establish the effectiveness of wound care.

Use the audit cycle presented (Figure 9.1) to design an audit that would demonstrate the effectiveness of wound care within the nursing team in Chettlesbridge.

You may wish to visit the web pages of the HCQIP (2009) dedicated to clinical audit to help with this task; the DH (2011a) may also be useful. You may have considered some of the questions below.

- Is our choice of topic relevant, justified?
- Will it be of interest to the team?

- Are any standards available: local wound care policies, national guidance?
- Do we agree with the standards? Is there anything we would want to add?
- How will we gather the data, patient records, would care charts, etc.?
- What are the results?
- Do we need to make any changes, set new standards?
- Do team members need additional training/education?
- Are there any other factors that need to be considered such as infection control processes, equipment and choice of dressings?
- When will we review any changes that we make?

 Discussion point

You could discuss clinical audit with your mentor in practice. Is there an audit tool for wound care?

Clinical audit vs research

There is sometimes a little confusion between what constitutes clinical audit and research. Essentially research is the pursuit and creation of new knowledge, concerned with determining best practice. Clinical audit, on the other hand, is about checking that we are applying the research, the best practice. The Royal College of Nursing outline the differences, which have been reproduced in Table 9.1.

In the scenario described above, a researcher may ask, 'What is the best way to manage wounds?' A team of nurses may use the research to ask 'are we managing wounds using the best practice guidance?'.

Chapter summary

This chapter has posed a series of questions that should help you to ensure the care you deliver is of high quality. It has considered the impact of nursing care on health outcomes for your patients. Specifically it has:

- demonstrated the need for identifying, evaluating and measuring outcomes of care;
- guided you to strategies that support a culture of continuous improvement in your work place;

Table 9.1 Differences between research and clinical audit

Research	Clinical audit
Adds new knowledge about what works or what doesn't.	Answers the question 'are we following best practice?'.
Aims to establish what is best practice.	Aims to improve practice.
Is designed so that it can be replicated so that the results are transferable to other similar groups.	Is specific and local to one patient group – the results are not transferable to other settings (although audit process may be of interest to wider audience and hence clinical audits are also published).
May involve allocating service users randomly to different treatment groups.	Never involves random allocation of service users to different treatment groups.
May involve the use of a placebo (a substance containing no medication, used especially in controlled experiments testing the efficacy of another substance such as a drug).	Never involves the use of a placebo.
May involve a completely new treatment.	Never involves a completely new treatment.

- introduced a framework to enable evidence-based practice;
- considered the role of clinical audit in ensuring good outcomes of care.

NMC Essential Skill Cluster (ESC)	ESC number
Care, Compassion and Communication	4, 5
Organizational Aspects of Care	10, 12
Infection Prevention and Control	
Nutrition and Fluid Management	
Medicines Management	

References

Aveyard, H. and Sharp, P. (2009) *A Beginner's Guide to Evidence Based Practice in Health and Social Care.* Maidenhead: Open University Press.

Burls, A. (2009) *What is Critical Appraisal?*, 2nd edn. http://www.medicine .ox.ac.uk/bandolier/painres/download/whatis/What_is_critical_appraisal.pdf (accessed 20 July 2011).

CASP (Critical Appraisal Skills Programme) (2011) *Find, Appraise, Act.* http:// www.casp-uk.net/homepage/ (accessed 20 July 2011).

Chapman, J., Bachard, D. and Hryka, S. (2011) Testing the sensitivity, specificity and feasibility of four risk assessment tools in a clinical setting. *Journal of Nursing Management*, 19: 133–42.

DH (Department of Health) (2010a) *Equity and Excellence: Liberating the NHS*. London: DH.

DH (2010b) *The NHS Constitution*. The NHS Belongs to Us All. http://www.nhs.uk/choiceintheNHS/Rightsandpledges/NHSConstitution/Documents/nhs-constitution-interactive-version-march-2010.pdf (accessed 20 July 2011).

DH (2010c) *The NHS Outcomes Framework 2011/12*. London: DH.

DH (2011a) *The Government's Response to the Recommendations in Front Line Care: The Report of the Prime Minister's Commission on the Future of Nursing and Midwifery in England*. http://www.dh.gov.uk/prod_consum_dh/groups/dh_digitalassets/documents/digitalasset/dh_125985.pdf (accessed 20 July 2011).

DH (2011b) *Transforming Community Services: Demonstrating and Measuring Achievement: Community Indicators for Quality Improvement*. http://www.dh.gov.uk/en/Publicationsandstatistics/Publications/PublicationsPolicyAndGuidance/DH_126110 (accessed 20 July 2011).

Gopee, N. and Galloway, J. (2009) *Leadership and Management in Healthcare*. London: Sage.

HCQIP (Healthcare Quality Improvement Partnership) (2009) *What is Clinical Audit?* http://www.hqip.org.uk/assets/Uploads/HQIP-What-is-Clinical-Audit-Nov-09.pdf (accessed 18 August 2011).

Leufer, T. and Cleary-Holdforth, J. (2009) Evidence-based practice: improving patient outcomes. *Nursing Standard*, 23(32): 35–9.

Lovallo, C., Rolandi, S., Rossetti, A.M. and Lusignani, M. (2009) Accidental falls in hospital inpatients: evaluation of sensitivity and specificity of two risk assessment tools. *Journal of Advanced Nursing*, 66(3): 690–6.

Manley, K., Watts, C., Cunningham, G. and Davies, J. (2011) Person centred care: principle of nursing practice. *Nursing Standard*, 25(31): 35–7.

Martin, V., Charlesworth, J. and Henderson, E. (2010) *Managing in Health and Social Care*. Oxford: Routledge.

Melnyk, B.M., Fineout-Overholt, E., Stillwell, S. and Williamson, K.M. (2010a) Evidence based practice step by step: the seven steps of evidence-based practice. *American Journal of Nursing*, 110(1): 51–3.

Melnyk, B.M., Fineout-Overholt, E., Stillwell, S. and Williamson, K.M. (2010b) Evidence based practice step by step: igniting a spirit of inquiry: an essential foundation for evidence-based practice. *American Journal of Nursing*, 109(11): 49–52.

Nightingale, F. (1854) *Notes on Matters Affecting Health, Efficiency, and Hospital Administration of the British Army*. London: Harrison and Sons.

NMC (Nursing Midwifery Council) (2008) *The Code: Standards of Conduct, Performance and Ethics for Nurses and Midwives*. London: NMC.

RCN (Royal College of Nursing) (2010) *Principles of Nursing Practice*. http://www.rcn.org.uk/development/practice/principles (accessed 20 July 2011).

World Health Organization (1998) *Health Promotion Glossary*. Geneva: World Health Organization.

Further reading

Burgess, R. (2010) *New Principles of Best Practice in Clinical Audit*, 2nd edn. Oxford: Radcliffe.

Useful websites

The NHS Information Centre www.ic.nhs.uk
The NHS Institute for Innovation and Improvement www.institute.nhs.uk

10 Health protection

Introduction

The aim of this chapter is for you to develop an understanding of the regulatory systems which are in place to promote human health and protect the population from harm. The chapter will discuss the role of health protection, and enable you to understand the various strategies that are used to protect against disease and promote improvements in health.

Learning outcomes

At the end of this chapter you should be able to:

- define the term health protection;
- identify the agencies and organizations involved in health protection;
- examine some of the strategies used to maintain population health;
- identify the role of the nurse in protecting health.

Health protection

The role of health protection has a long history and is best described as an approach 'to protect the community (or any part of the community) against infectious diseases and other dangers to health' (Health Protection Agency 2004).

This definition embraces the three main strands of health protection identified by Regan (1999) as: the prevention and control of communicable disease, non-infectious environmental hazards and health related emergency planning. This role is currently managed by the Health Protection Agency (http://www.hpa.org.uk/). The Health Protection Agency's role is to provide a cohesive approach to health protection through support and advice to the NHS, local authorities, emergency services and other organizations that have a public health responsibility.

The modern day threats to human health can be summarized under the following headings:

- an acute major incident due to climate change such as a natural disaster, radioactive leakage from a nuclear installation;
- a major food poisoning outbreak or food contamination;
- public accidents: train crash, acts of terrorism;
- acute and chronic health threats from industrial pollution;

- possible health hazards from new technology; genetically modified foods, telecommunications;
- developing new infectious diseases.

(Grey and Sarangi, in Orme et al. 2005: 108)

Questions

1. Think about some of the environmental catastrophes which have occurred in recent years. How have these impacted on the population's health?
2. Think about water, sanitation and food supplies. What are the risks to the population if these systems become damaged or contaminated in any way?
3. What do you know about the impact of air pollution on the public's health?
4. What measures are there in place to monitor and improve air quality?

The health impact of these modern day threats can impact at a local, national or global level. An outbreak of gastro-enteritis in a nursing home can be quickly contained, once the source of infection has been identified and appropriate treatment instigated. However, if we consider the complexity and distances of food transportation it is clear that should food become contaminated as in the Eschericia Coli 0104:04 outbreak in Germany in 2011 (*The Guardian* 2011) the risk to human health can escalate rapidly spreading across national and international boundaries and will necessitate international collaboration to bring the outbreak under control.

The success of health protection processes can only be achieved through robust collaboration between the different systems that identify, monitor and report health risk, and those who develop policies and organizational systems to protect human health (Grey and Sarangi cited in Orme et al. 2005).

Reflection

Can you identify everyday public activities which help to protect against widespread infection?

Think about public health messages which appear in the media. Infection control policies; food handling practices you may have observed when purchasing food.

What organizations can you think of that protect the public's health?

Have a look at some of the websites below to help you answer these questions.

Food handling http://www.food.gov.uk/foodindustry/regulation/hygleg/hygleginfo/foodhygknow/

Environment Agency http://www.environment-agency.gov.uk/

Air quality standards http://www.legislation.gov.uk/uksi/2010/1001/contents/made

In the last activity, you were asked to consider some of the strategies that have been put in place to protect human health. As we have already identified, health protection is a complex interplay between lots of organizations which are responsible for an array of different activities and is described by Downie et al. as: 'legal or fiscal controls, other regulations and policies, and voluntary codes of practices, aimed at the enhancement of positive health and the prevention of ill-health' (Downie et al. 1996: 52).

Health protection considers the wider political, legislative and social environment and aims to reduce exposure to health hazards and makes access to healthier choices easier. Indeed, in 2004, the Department of Health Report *Choosing Health: Making Healthy Choices Easier* (DH 2004), outlined the importance of joint working and collaboration between the political, legislative and social agencies in order to help people have greater access to healthy life choices.

Reflection

Consider some of the recent public health developments that have impacted on the whole population. You might like to look up some articles about obesity, smoking, air quality? Consider the issue and how much it costs the Nation in terms of helth care, money lost because of sickness. What other measures might be taken.

History demonstrates that the adoption of a behaviour change is often slow. If we consider the voluntary introduction of safety belt use or the strategies to reduce smoking, these strategies were successful up to a point, but as Maryon-Davis (2010) argues, some public health measures require state intervention to achieve optimum health benefit. If we consider 'making healthier choices easier', the smoking ban impacted on those exposed to passive smoking as well as restricting the behaviours of smokers. Indeed, research by Menzies and Lipworth (2006) has identified a significant reduction in lung inflammation, rhinitis and asthma in pub workers in Scotland as a direct result of the smoking ban.

These government interventions may appear to be divorced from the role of the community nurse. However, Downie et al. (1996) would argue that they are an essential component of public health and strengthen the day to day health promoting and health protecting activities which nurses undertake.

Downie et al.'s model describes three interlinking areas of activity that together promote and protect health. If we consider prevention of communicable disease, the health education element might involve nurses discussing flu vaccination with patients, production of leaflets and messages through the media. The disease prevention component will include a vaccination programme in which nurses will be key. The health protection component will include the licensing of appropriate vaccines to prevent against flu.

Reflection

Look at Downie et al.'s model and think about other areas of health protection and identify the different activities that might be undertaken at the different level to improve health.

Communicable diseases

The prevention of the spread of communicable disease is a key function of health protection and one particular area of health protection where community nurses have an influence, particularly in the administration of immunization.

Communicable diseases are infectious diseases that spread from person to person through air, water, food and human contact. They are numerous and include diseases such as influenza, hiv, polio, mumps, measles, chicken pox and salmonella.

The majority of work undertaken by health protection personnel to prevent and control the spread of communicable disease involves disease outbreak management. This is also known as communicable disease surveillance and involves the continuous monitoring of the frequency and distribution of disease. This will involve monitoring gastro-enteritis outbreaks in community hospitals, nursing homes and nurseries and food-borne outbreaks (food poisoning) which are managed in conjunction with the local environmental health department.

Communicable disease surveillance also identifies which infections are most likely to cause most illness, disability and mortality. This process also identifies which groups within the population are most at risk; for example young children, the elderly, those who are immune suppressed or have other physical conditions which make them more vulnerable if they contract certain diseases.

Certain diseases are 'notifiable' as they cause significant risk and harm to population health. When a doctor becomes aware of a suspected case of a notifiable disease in England and Wales, they have a statutory duty to notify a 'Proper Officer' in the local authorities under the Health Protection Notification Regulations (DH 2010). In some instances, the management of an outbreak may lead to immunization against the disease; for example in bacterial meningitis (Salisbury et al. 2006).

Immunization

Immunization is pivotal in preventing the spread of communicable disease and protecting the health of the whole population. According to the Health Protection Agency 'After clean water, vaccination is the most effective public health intervention in the world for saving lives and promoting good health' (Health Protection Agency 2004).

Immunization protects children and adults against harmful infections before they come into contact with them in the community. Immunization is usually given as an injection and describes the process of receiving the vaccine and becoming immune to the disease. Immunization invokes an immune response; this is achieved through the administration of small doses of an antigen, such as dead or weakened live viruses which are given to the individual to activate the immune system, or 'memory system'. When activated, the 'memory system' allows the body to react quickly and efficiently to future exposures.

The Joint Committee on Vaccination and Immunization (JCVI) is an independent expert advisory committee responsible for providing advice and scientific evidence to the UK health departments in the planning of immunization schedules for children, travel immunization programmes and older people. Once recommendations from JCVIs receive approval, they are funded centrally from government and vaccines are provided free to those who receive them.

Most immunization programmes are managed within primary care and community nurses have a key function in this. Childhood immunizations are usually given within GP surgeries as there is a payment attached to the immunization provision a practice may provide (Salisbury 2005).

Community nurses have a significant role in the prevention and control of communicable disease and the implementation of immunization programmes is one of the community nurse's key functions in controlling the spread of infectious disease. This role includes advising individuals about immunization, and administering vaccines as set down in the Department of Health's Green Book: *Immunisation Against Infectious Disease* (Salisbury et al. 2006). Health visitors, school nurses, practice nurses, district nurses and community staff nurses all have responsibility for ensuring certain sections of the population engage in immunization programmes.

 Questions

Have a look at the different immunization schedules by accessing the Department of Health website for immunization (http://www.dh.gov.uk/en/Publichealth/Immunisation/Vaccineupdate/index.htm) and identify which immunizations might be given to:

- Elizabeth and Evie Brown;
- Michael and Larry;
- Eileen, Mary and the twins.

Discuss with your mentor how individuals are contacted and informed about immunization. Who is responsible for giving the immunizations and where they might be given; i.e. a clinic, the home environment or a GP practice. Discuss the advice that is given when immunizations are given. How do you store vaccines safely? The Green Book is an excellent resource to find the answers to some of these questions.

Mary has 4-year-old twin boys, Peter and Simon. The boys are due to start school in September and Mary has to complete a health questionnaire for the school nursing services. She is asked to confirm the twins' immunization status. The boys were born on 17 November 2006 and have completed their preschool immunization programme.

Take a look at the immunization schedule for all pre-school children (http://www.nhs.uk/Planners/vaccinations/Pages/Vaccinationchecklist.aspx) and complete the immunization section of the health questionnaire (Table 10.1). The correct schedule can be found in the Appendix.

Table 10.1 Limestreet Primary School record of immunization

Limestreet Primary School Reception Year Entrants' Health Questionnaire
Record of Immunization

Name of Immunization	Date
2 Months	
3 Months	
4 Months	
12–13 Months	
3 Years and 4 Months	

Herd immunity

Immunization aims to achieve a level of herd immunity within a population. Herd immunity describes a form of immunity that occurs when a significant proportion of the population has been immunized to provide a level of protection for those who have not developed immunity to that specific disease. Different diseases require a different level of herd immunity to achieve this level of protection, and for most diseases this is about 95 per cent (John and Samuel 2000). The general rule is that if enough individuals are immunized with an effective vaccine against a specific disease, the spread of disease is likely to be disrupted and unimmunized individuals are at little or any risk of contracting the disease. If the level of herd immunity drops below a certain level then there is a risk that the disease can return. The MMR immunization is an example of this. Research by Dr Andrew Wakefield (Wakefield 1999) suggested there was a link between the MMR vaccine, autism and bowel disease. The research, which was later disproved, led to huge lack of public confidence in the MMR vaccine and the uptake rate, which needs to be at 90 per cent to achieve herd immunity, dropped significantly below this, resulting in outbreaks of mumps and measles within the population (Health Protection Agency 2008).

Community nurses are required to advise individuals and families about immunizations and need to understand the sound evidence base which supports immunization programmes as patients now have access to a large range of information, particularly taken from the Internet.

 Discussion points

- Discuss with your mentor where they find the evidence to support the questions patients may have about different vaccines.
- Elizabeth and Evie will due to have an influenza vaccine. How would you advise them?
- Can you identify any leaflets or information that are available for patients in your placements? Ask your mentor where these come from.

Chapter summary

In this chapter we have identified the types of activities that are undertaken to protect the population's health. We have considered the importance of the different strands of health protection, which might initially feel distant from the everyday work of a community nurse, but in reality affect us all, especially when things go wrong. These health protection strands include food safety legislation and measures to maintain clean water supplies and immunization programmes to protect the population from infectious disease. The nurse needs to be aware of these systems and processes and how they relate to the nurse's role in protecting human health.

NMC Essential Skill Cluster (ESC)	ESC number
Care, Compassion and Communication	1, 2, 3, 4, 5, 6, 7
Organizational Aspects of Care	9, 10, 11, 13, 15, 17, 18
Infection Prevention and Control	21, 24

References

DH (Department of Health) (2004) *Choosing Health: Making Healthy Choices Easier.* London: The Stationery Office.

DH (2010) *Guidance on the Health Protection (Notification) Regulations.* London: DH.

Downie, R.S., Tannahill, C. and Tannahill, A. (1996) *Health Promotion Model and Values*, 2nd edn. Oxford: Oxford University Press.

The Guardian (2011) *The Reason why this Deadly E coli Makes Doctors Shudder.* http://www.guardian.co.uk/commentisfree/2011/jun/05/deadly-ecoli-resistance-antibiotic-misuse (accessed 18 August 2011).

Health Protection Agency (2004) *Vaccination Immunisation.* http://www.hpa.org.uk/Topics/InfectiousDiseases/InfectionsAZ/VaccinationImmunisation/ (accessed 18 August 2011).

Health Protection Agency (2008) *MMR Vaccine Plea as Measles Continues to Spread.* http://www.hpa.org.uk/ProductsServices/LocalServices/NorthWest/North WestNewsArchive/nwest081103MMRvaccineplea/ (accessed 1 September 2011).

John, T.J. and Samuel, R. (2000) Herd immunity and herd effect: new insights and definitions. *European Journal of Epidemiology*, 16(7): 601–6.

Maryon-Davis, A. (2010) *Healthy Nudges: When the Public Want Change and the Politicians Don't Know It.* London: Faculty of Public Health.

Menzies, D. and Lipworth, B. (2006) Respiratory Symptoms, Pulmonary Function, and Markers of Inflammation Among Bar Workers Before and After a Legislative Ban on Smoking in Public Places. *JAMA*, 297(4): 359–60.

NMC (Nursing Midwifery Council) (2008) *The Code: Standards of Conduct, Performance and Ethics for Nurses and Midwives.* London: NMC.

NMC (2010) *Essential Skills Clusters and Guidance for their Use.* London: NMC.

Orme, J., Powell, J., Taylor, P., Harrison, T. and Grey, M. (2005) *Public Health Policy for the 21st Century: New Perspectives on Policy, Participation and Practice.* Maidenhead: Open University Press.

Regan, M. (1999) Health protection in the next millennium from tactics to strategy. *Journal of Epidemiology and Community Health*, 53: 517–18.

Salisbury, D. (2005) Development of immunization policy and its implementation in the United Kingdom. *Health Affairs*, 24(3): 744–54.

Salisbury, D., Ramsay, M. and Noakes, K. (eds) (2006) *Immunisation Against Infectious Disease.* London: The Stationery Office.

Wakefield, A. (1999) MMR and autism. *The Lancet*, 354(9282): 949–50.

Further reading

Health Protection Agency www.hpa.org.uk

11 Community nursing practice – becoming a registered nurse

Introduction

This chapter explores the issues related to the transition from being a student nurse to becoming an accountable, registered practitioner. The chapter will introduce you to some ideas that will help to support your development as a qualified nurse who can affect, manage and maintain change in patient care within a professional, ethical and legal framework. The chapter will consider the development of your confidence, competence and self-awareness as a future leader of your profession. The development of skills and an understanding of clinical leadership will be introduced. Personal development plans will be introduced as tools for recording your successes in practice and identifying areas for improvement to ensure continuous development.

This chapter will cover:

- developing competence, confidence and self-awareness;
- developing skills in leadership;
- career planning.

During this chapter you will be invited to consider your individual learning needs. You will be provided with an opportunity to develop a personal development plan (PDP) at the end of the chapter, by reflecting on your learning needs for the transition you will make from student to registered nurse.

The transition from student to registered practitioner is the subject of much nursing literature. There is a focus on the development of competence and confidence and in particular the added professional accountability that registration brings.

The development of the PDP will help you to consider the strategies you may adopt once qualified in recording the impact learning has on practice. Registered nurses have to complete 450 hours of practice and 35 hours of learning activity in a three year period to remain on the register as a nurse (NMC 2008b). You may be asked to demonstrate how you have maintained contemporary practice. You should be able to articulate how your learning has informed your practice.

The themes raised in this chapter should be read within the context of the Nursing and Midwifery Council (NMC) Code of Conduct for Nurses and Midwives (NMC 2008a). The code states: 'As a professional, you are personally accountable for actions and omissions in your practice and must always be able to justify your decisions.'

Learning outcomes

At the end of this chapter you should be able to:

- acknowledge the importance of leadership in nursing for quality care;
- recognize your strengths and areas for development;
- use a personal development plan to articulate your learning and how this has impacted on your professional practice.

Developing competence and confidence

Development of competence

During your pre-registration education you will have been prepared to meet the standards required of registered nurses by the NMC. These standards are set out in the standards of proficiency for pre-registration nursing education (NMC 2010). Meeting these standards ensures you are competent to carry out the role of a registered nurse. Your competence will have been assessed in practice by your mentors during your nursing education. There should be no question that you are competent to practise as a registered nurse at the point of registration. The post-registration period should be focused on the acquisition of specific clinical competencies that you may not have been exposed to during your education programme.

While newly qualified nurses are considered competent, several studies suggest that a lack of confidence is common in newly qualified nurses (Clark and Holmes 2007; Roberts and Johnson 2009; Higgins et al. 2010). This lack of confidence has also been highlighted by several studies considered in a systematic review by Higgins et al. (2010). Lack of confidence was described in the review by some studies as short lived; one study reviewed suggesting that confidence was acquired over time and was not something that could be taught. The majority of papers reviewed highlighted an increase in responsibility and accountability as a major stressor in the transition to registered nurse. The studies reviewed also found that newly qualified nurses had an unrealistic expectation of their new role and the reality of practice.

 Discussion point

When you are on placement, talk to the newly qualified nurses. Discuss your expectations with your mentor.

How does the reality of practice differ from expectation? How might this impact on your confidence?

The importance of learning in the development of confidence is discussed by Roberts and Johnson (2009). It is suggested that the more confident a student is perceived to be the more they will be allowed to do. For students, being allowed to do more is viewed as evidence that they are learning, perhaps indicating that the development of confidence and competence are linked. This supports the findings of an earlier study by Clark and Holmes (2007). The exploration of the development of newly qualified nurses suggested a link between the development of competence and increased confidence. Confidence for newly qualified nurses was increased when there was an acceptance into the team which seemed to be determined by the ability to perform specific nursing tasks. It would seem from the studies discussed above that the development of confidence occurs alongside the achievement of competence.

It could be said that working in the community setting requires a higher level of confidence than in a hospital setting. As we have seen in earlier chapters community nurses are mostly working alone. There may be a team of people to support you in your role but ultimately when visiting a patient in their own home it is you that the patient is relying on to know what you are doing. Being confident in your approach will help patients to be confident in you. The Department of Health publication *Confidence in Caring* (DH 2008a) states that the creation of confidence for patients can be displayed at an organizational, team and individual level. 'At the individual level, confidence can be created when patients see that individuals have the skills to do the job and the will to provide the level of care that patient wants' (DH 2008a: 6).

Developing confidence through preceptorship

A period of preceptorship is recognized as an essential part of ensuring a smooth transition from student to staff nurse. This is supportive of the findings of a review by Robinson and Griffiths (2009) that preceptorship was regarded as having a key role in assisting the transition from student to registered nurse.

Nurses working in the NHS are subject to agenda for change pay system; it was introduced in 2004 to provide an improved career framework and fairer pay structure for all staff in the NHS. In terms of pay, agenda for change provides a pay structure in bands, each band having several pay points. Staff can progress through the pay points annually provided they have met the performance indicators. Newly qualified professional staff, including nurses, have the opportunity to accelerate through two pay points during the first year in post. This 12 month period is defined by the NHS Staff Council as preceptorship (NHS Staff Council 2011). The importance of preceptorship for newly qualified health professionals has been recognized by the Department of Health who in 2010 published a preceptorship framework (DH 2010b). The framework defines preceptorship as:

> A period of structured transition for the newly registered practitioner during which he or she will be supported by a preceptor, to develop their confidence as an autonomous professional, refine skills, values and behaviours and to continue on their journey of life-long learning.
>
> (DH 2010b: 11)

The work of Albert Bandura (1977) can be drawn upon in the consideration of the development of confidence during this preceptorship period for newly qualified nurses. Bandura (1994) describes self-efficacy as an individual's belief that they can succeed. The degree of self-efficacy can determine how goals, tasks and challenges are approached. Four foundations for self-efficacy have been defined:

- *Mastery experiences* When tasks are performed successfully a strong sense of self-efficacy is developed, however failing to perform successfully can be demoralizing and self-efficacy diminished.
- *Social modelling* Seeing other people succeed increases the belief that an individual can succeed.
- *Social persuasion* Encouragement from others that success is achievable supports 'can do' behaviours and the belief that success is achievable.
- *Psychological responses* Stress is minimized by responding positively to challenges.

While Bandura emphasizes that confidence and self-efficacy are not the same thing, it could be argued that self-efficacy can lead to the development of self-confidence. The attributes of an effective preceptor have been defined by the DH (2010b) to include:

- giving constructive feedback – 'social persuasion';
- setting goals and assessing competency – 'mastery experiences';
- being an effective and inspirational role model and demonstrating professional values, attitude and behaviours – 'social modelling';
- facilitating problem solving – 'psychological responses'.

It would seem that a well prepared preceptor and practice settings that provide a supportive environment can provide the foundations for the development of self-efficacy.

 Reflection

Take some time to reflect on each of the foundations of self-efficacy above and ask yourself:

- What have been my successes so far?
- What practices do I observe that achieve good outcomes?
- Do others tell me I am performing well?
- Am I positive, how do I cope with stress?

Record your reflections in your reflective journal.

Believing in yourself could be the key to developing confidence in your practice. Use your PDP to:

- record your successes;
- look for challenges, identify areas for development and make a plan to meet your goals;
- be committed to personal and professional development: set short-, medium- and longer-term goals;
- identify your stressors and strategies to minimize the negative effect of stress.

Emotional intelligence

Emotional intelligence provides a way in which individual behaviours and the impact of those behaviours on others can be understood. It could be argued that emotional intelligence put simply is about:

- understanding yourself, your goals, intentions, responses and your behaviour;
- understanding others, and their feelings.

Emotional intelligence has been popularized by the work of Daniel Goleman since the publication of his book *Emotional Intelligence* in 2009. Goleman defines emotional intelligence as having five domains:

1. knowing your emotions;
2. managing your own emotions;
3. motivating yourself;
4. recognizing and understanding other people's emotions;
5. managing relationships, managing the emotions of others.

Goleman has identified five elements of emotional intelligence:

1. self-awareness
2. self-regulation
3. motivation
4. empathy
5. social skills.

Goleman believes that by developing our emotional intelligence we can become more productive and successful at what we do, while helping others to be more productive and successful too. Nurses have a moral and professional obligation through the Code of Conduct (NMC 2008a) to make every effort to improve the way we work. It is hoped that by exploring concepts such as emotional intelligence relationships with colleagues, patients and their carers can be supportive, balanced and therapeutic. According to Goleman, emotional intelligence is also an essential element of leadership. His research suggests successful leaders all possess a high level of emotional intelligence.

The role of emotional intelligence in nursing is generally supported by Bulmer Smith et al. (2009). This review concludes that while there is evidence to suggest that emotional intelligence has an influence on nursing practice, further research is required to determine the importance of this concept in nursing. Consideration of whether emotional intelligence is needed for leadership is made through a series of academic letters by Antonakis et al. (2009), providing an alternative view of this popular concept.

Leadership

Leadership in nursing is the subject of much debate. There is a plethora of books, articles and research focused on the subject. The publication by Curtis et al. (2011a) provides a concise introduction to leadership in nursing. While there is much written about nursing leadership, it has been suggested that little literature exists that specifically examines leadership in community nursing (Kean et al. 2011).

Government policy has recently focused on the need for clinical leadership in the drive to improve the quality of experience, care and outcomes for patients. Clinical leadership was considered throughout Lord Darzi's review of the NHS in 2008 *High Quality Care for All* (DH 2008b). The Prime Minister's Commission on the Future of Nursing and Midwifery in England (2009) also put nurses (and midwives) at the centre of health leadership. Clinical leadership viewed as central to continuous improvement and delivery of high quality, safe and effective care. Leadership continues to feature as a constituent in new Government policy, although in the White Paper *Equity and Excellence: Liberating the NHS* (DH 2010a) leadership in commissioning seems to be the focus for driving improvement.

Leadership in community nursing

The Queen's Nursing Institute (QNI) (2009) recognized leadership in community nursing as being essential to the transformation that is required to ensure those nursed at home continue to receive the best quality care. A campaign launched in 2011 (QNI 2011) reinforces the need for the right nurse with the right skills and while this campaign is focused on clinical skills it is clear that clinical leadership is imperative in ensuring patients in their own homes receive the right care by nurses equipped with specific skills and knowledge. As well as ensuring clinical excellence, Haycock-Stuart et al. (2010) suggests that community nursing leaders need to develop competencies in strategic and political leadership.

The importance of nursing leadership has been highlighted as an important element in achieving key recommendations for the transformation on nursing practice (National Academy of Sciences 2011). Although the consideration in this report is on nursing in the United States of America, Jasper (2011) observes the message for nursing everywhere.

Leadership or management

While development in leadership and management may seem to be the domain of qualified, experienced nurses, the NMC (2010) require all student nurses to achieve competency in leadership and management. Gopee and Galloway (2009) provide a useful summary of the different theories and styles of management. Management in health care can be defined as 'a team of appropriately qualified individuals who engage in multiple activities aimed at achieving the goals of the organisation effectively and efficiently' (Gopee and Galloway 2009: 29).

The processes of management have been described by many theorists, and what managers do is the subject of much debate. The traditional interpretation of the activities of managers has been described as:

- planning
- organizing
- coordinating
- leading.

This chapter will focus on the activity of leading and nurses as leaders. Leadership will be discussed as the way in which management activities are performed and achieved.

Kean et al. (2011) recognize the confusion that can arise when discussing leadership and leaders, and while this research is focused on the notion of 'followers' in relation to leadership the authors make an interesting differentiation between 'leadership' and 'leaders'. They suggest the differences can be defined by considering leadership as a process, and being a leader defined by the 'characteristics and behaviours of individuals'. This is perhaps a useful distinction to draw when considering the development of leadership skills and abilities for nurses.

What is leadership?

The competencies required suggest that as a newly qualified nurse you should have competence in both being a 'leader' and 'leadership' as defined above. The ultimate purpose of leadership in nursing is to ensure the best outcomes of care and the best possible experience for patients. The leadership and management competencies required by the NMC (2010) would necessitate the acquisition of skills and knowledge in the following:

- delegating and supervising care;
- prioritizing care;
- coordination of care;
- planning and organizing;
- continuous evaluation of care;
- managing risk;
- acting as a change agent;
- working effectively with others across organizational and professional boundaries.

While many of these skills have been discussed in earlier chapters of this book, the exploration of management and leadership theory may support the development of associated skills and knowledge that will support the implementation of such activities in practice. Theories of leadership are abundant and much has been written about the qualities of leaders and how to perform leadership. Northouse (2010) offers several perspectives from which leadership in nursing could be explored. He describes what leadership is:

- *'Leadership is a trait'*
  Trait theory is one of the earlier theories of leadership, the premise being 'leaders are born not made'; 'great man' theory; leaders have unique, special characteristics.
- *'Leadership is ability'*
  As well as leadership being a natural ability as above, it is something that can be learned; people have the capacity to develop as leaders.

In nursing the development of leadership ability begins during pre-registration education. The impact of leadership training and education has been explored by Curtis et al. (2011b) who suggest that where leadership education is integrated with nursing and not taught within the context of management, it has a positive influence on the development of leadership skills.

- *'Leadership is a skill'*
  Development of competence in carrying out responsibilities and tasks assumes anyone can develop in leadership. Many different theorists have identified different competencies/skills/attributes of leaders, some of which will be considered later in this chapter.

For newly qualified nurses, competencies are set out in the standards for pre-registration nursing education, Section 2 Standards for Competence (NMC 2010).

- *'Leadership is a behaviour'*
  This concerns what leaders do and how they behave when they are in a leadership role. Leadership behaviour is often described as:
  - *Autocratic* The leader holds the decision-making power and is able to punish or reward team members.
  - *Democratic* All members of a team are encouraged by the leader to participate in decision making.
  - *Laissez-faire* The leader makes a conscious decision to pass the decision making to other team members.

- *'Leadership is a relationship'*
  Leadership is considered as dependent on the relationship between the leader and the follower, and not characteristics of the leader. This relationship is not influenced by position and supports development of leaders regardless of formal titles.

In the context of health care, Howatson-Jones (2004) explores the concept of 'servant leadership'. She suggests that serving the followers, needs benefits practice by strengthening the relationship between leaders and followers. This seems to support the notion above that leadership is a relationship.

- *'Leadership is an influence process'*
  Leaders influence others to set and achieve desired goals together. A similar definition to the latter has also been provided by Mullins (2010) who defines leadership as simply: 'a relationship through which one person influences the behaviour or actions of other people'.

In health care a transformational leadership style has been considered appropriate for health and is supportive of this view of leadership.

Transformational leadership

This has been discussed as a leadership approach for nursing (Jasper and Jumaa 2005; Hunter 2007; Gopee and Galloway 2009) merging the goals, desires and values of followers and leaders. Leaders inspire, motivate and encourage others to develop leadership, promoting independence and innovation.

Transactional leadership

This is an alternative approach to leadership, which has been described as the leader directing the team to achieve stated goals, interested in 'getting the job done'. While this is perhaps more reminiscent of the more traditional management styles, it could be argued that there is still a place for this type of leadership. In nursing this could be applied to delegating, managing risk, prioritizing, etc. Much like the description of autocratic leaders, it would seem that in nursing this approach is inappropriate, however in some situations this may be exactly the approach that is required.

Action-centred leadership

This is an approach developed in the 1980s by John Adair that is concerned with the relationship between the 'task', the 'team' and the 'individual'. It is depicted as three overlapping circles. Adair recognized that the most important element was the task. Attention to the team needs requires team building skills. Individuals' needs have to be identified and the leader must have an understanding of what motivates individual team members. The leader must ensure that the task is completed, the team are functioning and all individuals' needs are met. The leader's focus may shift between attending to the task, team or individual needs. Therefore the leader has to be continually monitoring each element and diverting their attention according to need (Adair 2010).

Situational or contingency theory

This type of leadership assumes that external factors determine the way in which leadership is carried out. Each situation will require a different approach; this requires the leaders to be flexible and have knowledge of the different approaches and which is best suited to what type of situation. The situation determines the leader's actions and the way the team functions.

 Questions

Can you think of an example of where it may be appropriate to adopt an autocratic style to leadership?

You may have thought about emergency situations – a cardiac arrest, a fire, a major incident – as situations where autocratic leadership should be adopted. In these situations the team needs to know what to do and each team member should be assigned specific tasks that the leader knows they are capable of carrying out precisely.

In what type of situations might it be best to adopt a more democratic approach to leadership?

Situations that require a more democratic approach may be utilized when a change is needed, for example when new evidence for practice has emerged, or an incident has occurred. The leader involves all the team members in the decision making, promoting creative and innovative thinking. The leader is motivating and supportive, all team members are included and views listened to and ideas nurtured.

Leadership continuum

In the 1950s Tannenbaum and Schmidt (1958) developed a model that considered leadership/management along a continuum. At one end of the continuum is the leader or manager who 'tells'; team members are expected to do exactly what the leader expects. At the other end of the continuum the leader or manager consults with team members, is collaborative and shared decision making is achieved. In between the 'telling' and 'collaborating' are five levels of 'freedom':

1. Tells – team members are expected to do exactly what the leader expects.
2. Sells – the leader explains decisions but does not expect any discussion.
3. Discusses – decisions are presented and questions invited.
4. Negotiates – a proposed decision is presented which is subject to change following discussion.
5. Consults – a problem is presented and ideas shared and discussed prior to a decision being made by the leader.

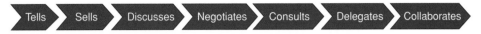

Figure 11.1 The Tannenbaum and Schmidt model

6. Delegates – decisions can be made by the team members and the leader defines the limits.
7. Collaborates – the leader enables the team or individual to act independently, to make decisions. The leader makes it known in advance that they support independent decision making. The leader may or may not include themselves as part of the team.

The Tannenbaum and Schmidt model is often depicted as a simple graph or table (see Figure 11.1). The ideal is that the leader moves from 'telling' to 'collaborating'. It should be said however that a team may not develop in this way and the leader may have to revert to telling at some stages and in some situations. We will come back to this model later in the chapter in relation to the delegation of nursing care.

 Reflection

Take a moment to think about the leaders and styles of leadership you may have seen in practice.

Have you experienced any of the types of leadership described above? How has your experience influenced the way in which you may develop as a leader and in your leadership role?

Leadership qualities

Considering the above definitions and approaches to leadership, it would seem there are certain behaviours and qualities that could be applied to leaders.

A leadership framework has been developed that outlines key aspects of leadership development for NHS employers and employees (National Leadership Council 2011). The framework is made up of seven domains, each with identified elements of effectiveness that support development within that domain.

One of the competencies outlined by the National Leadership Framework (2011) above is that of delegating and supervising care. Section 29 of the code (NMC 2008a) makes it clear that: 'You must establish that anyone you delegate care to is able to carry out your instructions'. Additional guidance stresses that as a registered nurse, you must ensure that:

- any individual that you delegate a task to is able to carry out your instruction;
- the task is completed to the required standard;
- all those persons you are responsible for are supervised and supported.

So not only you are accountable to the NMC for your own actions and omissions but in the case of a delegated task, those of others.

You can begin to explore your leadership and management qualities and the approach you might take as a leader by looking at the processes involved in the delegation and the supervision of others. Using the Tannenbaum and Schmidt leadership continuum consider each level of 'freedom' in relation to delegating a nursing task to another.

 Questions

1. What sort of tasks would require a telling approach to delegation?
2. What situations might you adopt a more consultative approach?
3. In what circumstances would you be confident to adopt a collaborative approach to delegation?

Possible answers to questions 1–3 are as follows:

1. You may have considered the case when someone is undertaking a task that is new to them. Precise instruction is required, with no ambiguity, the task to be undertaken within a clear set of guidelines, requirements for feedback clear.
2. You could have considered a case where you have a patient that may require some intervention that a member of the team has unique experience. You may discuss/negotiate/consult about the problem with the individual and use the information to support your decision making.
3. You may have considered the very experienced individual who you are able to ask to visit a patient for the first time such as the visit to Mrs Brown discussed in Chapters 3 and 7 earlier in the book. The individual would have to make an assessment and decide on a treatment option independently.

You may also have considered broader issues like local policies and procedures, training and education undertaken, the level of risk, etc.

Managing a caseload

This book has offered opportunities for you to consider concepts and develop knowledge and understanding of the specific skills that are required and has asked you to consider specific issues related to working in the community. This chapter has focused on the way in which management tasks are completed; how effective leadership can achieve the management tasks required. Earlier in this chapter management tasks were defined. Three of these tasks, planning, organizing and coordinating are essential skills needed for managing a caseload.

In earlier chapters you have considered many different factors that may influence how patients are cared for in community settings. Working with others and managing the assessment, care planning and evaluation of care all require the skills and knowledge presented in this chapter. How are the skills, knowledge and understanding applied to managing a caseload?

Managing the patients in Chettlesbridge

Consider the following scenarios for the patients that live in Chettlesbridge:

Michael has diabetes and while Larry is in hospital will need morning and evening doses of Insulin administered. You have had a call this morning from Joanne asking you to visit as his blood sugar reading was abnormally high and he seemed unwell.

Larry has been referred from the local hospital. He has had his heart surgery and requires an assessment visit today.

Mrs Brown's skin tear on her ankle has been regularly dressed following her fall. The wound has been taking longer to heal than anticipated. The report yesterday from Susan the community support worker suggests the wound may be developing into an ulcer.

Essie has become terminal and has required visits for symptom control. She has been visited every other day. Recently she has been experiencing difficulty with pain management and nausea. The GP has prescribed her analgesic and antiemetic medication to be administered subcutaneously. A syringe driver is required.

Eileen has called today requesting a visit as she is experiencing an exacerbation of her Chronic Obstructive Pulmonary Disease (COPD) and feels she may be developing a chest infection.

The team members that are available on duty today are as follows:

Jane – working 08.00 to 16.30

Paula – working 06.00 to 13.00

Joanne – working 08.00 to 20.00

Use the information presented above and throughout the book to consider the following questions.

 Questions

How would you go about deciding who was visited by when and by whom? What factors would need to be taken into consideration when making decisions? It is apparent that all the patients needed a visit today. It is important to consider the skills and experience of the individual team members. You may ask yourself:

- What competencies are required?

You need a team member competent in wound assessment, COPD, diabetes, perhaps a prescriber and someone who has initiated subcutaneous syringe driver therapy.

- Which team members have the required competence?

You will need to know who in the team has had the required training and has up to date knowledge and skills.

- What time are the visits required? Who will be on duty?

Check the off duty – has anyone called in sick? How long will each visit take, will the team member be able to complete the visit and leave work on time?

- Where do the patients live, how much travelling is involved? Can you divide the visits by geography? Does one team member have the competence to manage Michael's, Larry's and Eileen's problems?

You need to take account of the cost of the visit, and who can carry it out. For example if only Joanne can initiate the syringe driver therapy and needs to visit Eileen, how long will it take to get from one side of Chettlesbridge to the other?

- Are there any further referrals required? Who else may be able to visit these patients?

There may be a community matron in the team who is involved in Eileen's care. You may have access to a diabetes specialist, a wound care therapist, etc.

You may use these questions during your community placement to guide your learning and development.

 Reflection

Think about your development so far in respect of the knowledge, understanding and skills that would be required to manage the care of the residents of Chettlesbridge. Look back at the case scenarios and associated information presented in earlier chapters and remind yourself of the care required by each family.

The framework in Figure 11.2 is an example of how you could record your successes so far, your personal development/learning needs and the outcome of your learning. You could complete a PDP for each of the chapters in this book.

Personal development need	Action and resources needed	Review date

What was my prior knowledge/success so far?		
How has my new learning improved my knowledge/understanding		

What changes will be evident in my practice as a result of my learning and improved understanding?	Previous related practice	Enhanced practice

Figure 11.2 Personal development plan
Source: Framework adapted by Sarah Pye with kind permission from a framework presented to students at Canterbury Christ Church University by Annaliese Woods.

Career planning

The Department of Health have published a Nursing Career Framework (DH 2011) in which it outlines potential career pathways for nurses. The pathways are identified as:

1. mental health and psychosocial care;
2. supporting long-term care;
3. first contact, access and urgent care;
4. acute and critical care;
5. family and public health.

Throughout this book it is hoped that you have developed an understanding that community nursing and the diverse settings of care provide ample opportunity to develop your nursing career. The pathways identified by the Department of Health clearly outline career pathways for community nurses in the long-term care, first contact and family and public health pathways. The framework identifies the sort of job roles within the pathways that nurses may undertake, taking account of level of experience and academic achievement.

The career prospects for community nurses are exciting, with the identification of clinical roles including:

- staff nurse
- specialist nurse
- nurse practitioner and
- consultant nurse.

For nurse with an interest in education and research there are roles such as:

- research nurse
- lecturer or
- professor.

For those nurses who favour a management career roles include:

- team leader
- community matron and
- director of public health.

During your time as a student nurse you will be exposed to many different aspects of nursing. In your first post as a staff nurse and subsequent years as a registered nurse you will undoubtedly develop an interest in a particular aspect of nursing. Developing skills and knowledge in clinical and then strategic and political leadership require the development of an inquisitive nature that will ensure constant reconsideration of your practice. Keeping a PDP that encourages reflection, recognizes successes, identifies areas of learning needs and provides a strategy for continual development will help to support your career planning.

Chapter summary

This chapter has introduced you to strategies that may support your transition from a student nurse to a registered nurse. In particular this chapter has:

- demonstrated that the successful progression from student to registrant relies on the development of confidence and leadership skills as well as clinical competence, knowledge and skills;
- identified strategies and processes that are available to you and to potential employers to facilitate successful, effective integration to a nursing team.

It is hoped that you may use the PDP template to record your learning and identify future development needs. It is a tool that should demonstrate your successes as well. It can be used to help you consider how theory informs practice.

NMC Essential Skill Cluster (ESC)	ESC number
Organizational Aspects of Care	12, 13, 14, 15, 16, 17

References

Adair, J. (2010) *Effective Leadership: How to be a Successful Leader.* London: Pan Macmillan.

Antonakis, J., Ashkanasy, N. and Dasborough, M. (2009) Does leadership need emotional intelligence? *The Leadership Quarterly,* (20): 247–61.

Bandura, A. (1977) Self-efficacy: toward a unifying theory of behavioral change. *Psychological Review,* 84: 191–215.

Bandura, A. (1994) Self-efficacy. In V.S. Ramachandran (ed.) *Encyclopedia of Human Behavior.* New York: Academic Press.

Bulmer Smith, K., Profetto-McGrath, J. and Cummings, G. (2009) Emotional intelligence and nursing: an integrative literature review. *International Journal of Nursing Studies,* 46: 1624–36.

Clark, T. and Holmes, S. (2007) Fit for practice? An exploration of the development of newly qualified nurses using focus groups. *International Journal of Nursing Studies,* 44: 1210–20.

Curtis, E., Vries, J., Fintan, K. and Sheerin, F. (2011a) Developing leadership in nursing: exploring core factors. *British Journal of Nursing,* 20(5): 306–9.

Curtis, E., Vries, J., Fintan, K. and Sheerin, F. (2011b) Developing leadership in nursing: the impact of education and training. *British Journal of Nursing,* 20(6): 344–52.

DH (Department of Health) (2008a) *Confidence in Caring: A Framework for Best Practice.* London: Department of Health. http://www.dh.gov.uk/prod_consum _dh/groups/dh_digitalassets/@dh/@en/documents/digitalasset/dh_086388.pdf (accessed 11 May 2011).

DH (2008b) *High Quality Care for All: NHS Next Stage Review Final Report.* London: Department of Health. http://www.dh.gov.uk/en/Publicationsandstatistics/ Publications/PublicationsPolicyAndGuidance/DH_085825 (accessed 26 May 2011).

DH (2010a) *Equity and Excellence: Liberating the NHS.* London: Department of Health. http://www.dh.gov.uk/en/Publicationsandstatistics/Publications/ PublicationsPolicyAndGuidance/DH_117353 (accessed 26 May 2011).

DH (2010b) *Preceptorship Framework for Newly Registered Nurses, Midwives and Allied Health Professionals.* London: Department of Health. http://www.dh.gov.uk/ prod_consum_dh/groups/dh_digitalassets/@dh/@en/@abous/documents/ digitalasset/dh_114116.pdf (accessed 11 May 2011).

DH (2010c) *National Leadership Council Vision: Outstanding Leadership at Every Level of the NHS.* London: National Leadership Council.

DH (2011) *Modernising Nursing Careers: Nursing Career Framework.* http://www.dh.gov.uk/prod_consum_dh/groups/dh_digitalassets/documents/digitalasset/dh_108369.pdf (accessed 20 July 2011).

Goleman, D. (2009) *Emotional Intelligence: Why it Can Matter More than IQ.* London: Bloomsbury.

Gopee, N. and Galloway, J. (2009) *Leadership and Management in Healthcare.* London: Sage.

Haycock-Stuart, E., Baggaley, S., Kean, S. and Carson, M. (2010) Understanding leadership in community nursing in Scotland. *Community Practitioner*, 83(7): 24–8.

Higgins, G., Spencer, R.L. and Kane, R. (2010) A systematic review of the experiences and perceptions of the newly qualified nurse in the United Kingdom. *Nurse Education Today*, 30: 499–508.

Howatson-Jones, I.L. (2004) The servant leader. *Nursing Management*, 11(3): 20–4.

Hunter, D. (ed.) (2007) *Managing For Health.* London: Routledge.

Jasper, M. (2011) Editorial: Experiences of leadership in nursing management. *Journal of Nursing Management*, 19(4): 419–20.

Jasper, M. and Jumaa, M. (2005) *Effective Health Care Leadership.* Oxford: Blackwell.

Kean, S., Haycock-Stuart, E., Baggaley, S. and Carson, M. (2011) Followers and the co-construction of leadership. *Journal of Nursing Management*, 19(4): 507–16.

Mullins, L. (2010) *Management and Organisational Behaviour*, 9th edn. Harlow: Pearson.

(The) National Academy of Sciences (2011) *The Future of Nursing: Leading Change, Advancing Health.* Washington: The National Academies Press. http://www.nap.edu/openbook.php?record_id=12956 (accessed 26 May 2011).

NHS Staff Council (2011) *NHS Terms and Conditions of Service Handbook. Amendment Number 24 Pay Circular (AforC) 3/2011.* http://www.nhsemployers.org/SiteCollectionDocuments/AfC_tc_of_service_handbook_fb.pdf (accessed 11 May 2011).

National Leadership Council (2011) *National Leadership Framework.* Leeds: National Leadership Council.

Northouse, P. (2010) *Leadership: Theory and Practice*, 5th edn. London: Sage.

NMC (Nursing and Midwifery Council) (2008a) *The Code: Standards of Conduct, Performance and Ethics for Nurses and Midwives.* London: Nursing and Midwifery Council. http://www.nmc-uk.org/Documents/Standards/nmcTheCodeStandardsofConductPerformanceAndEthicsForNursesAndMidwives_LargePrintVersion.pdf (accessed 11 May 2011).

NMC (2008b) *The Prep Handbook* [online]. http://www.nmc-uk.org/Documents/Standards/nmcPrepHandbook.pdf (accessed 1 May 2011).

NMC (2010) *Standards of Proficiency for Pre-registration Nursing Education.* London: Nursing and Midwifery Council. http://www.nmc-uk.org/Educators/Standards-for-education/Standards-of-proficiency-for-pre-registration-nursing-education/ (accessed 11 May 2011).

Queen's Nursing Institute (2011) A position statement: nursing people in their own homes – key issues for the future of care. London: QNI.

Queen's Nursing Institute (2009) *2020 Vision: Focusing on the Future of District Nursing.* London: Queen's Nursing Institute.

Report by the Prime Minister's Commission of the Future of Nursing and Midwifery in England (2009) *Front Line Care.* London: Prime Minister's Commission of the Future of Nursing and Midwifery.

Roberts, D. and Johnson, M. (2009) Editorial. Newly qualified nurses: competence or confidence? *Nurse Education Today,* 29(5): 467–8.

Robinson, S. and Griffiths, P. (2009) *Scoping Review. Preceptorship for Newly Qualified Nurses: Impacts, Facilitators and Constraints.* London: National Nursing Research Unit King's College London. http://www.kcl.ac.uk/content/1/c6/05/06/70/PreceptorshipReview.pdf (accessed 11 May 2011).

Science Direct http://www.sciencedirect.com/science/article/pii/S0260691709000033 (accessed 26 May 2011).

Tannenbaum, R. and Schmidt, W.H. (1958) How to choose a leadership pattern. *Harvard Business Review,* 36: 95–101.

Further reading

Barr, J. and Dowling, L. (2008) *Leadership in Health Care.* London: Sage.

Bishop, V. (2009) *Leadership for Nursing and Allied Health Professionals.* Maidenhead: Open University Press.

Department of Health (2008) *A High Quality Workforce: NHS Next Stage Review.* London: Department of Health.

Lauder, W., Watson, R., Topping, K. et al. (2008) An evaluation of fitness for practice curricula: self-efficacy, support and self-reported competence in preregistration student nurses and midwives. *Journal of Clinical Nursing,* 17: 1858–67.

Martin, V., Charlesworth, J. and Henderson, E. (2010) *Managing in Health and Social Care.* 2nd edn. Abingdon: Routledge.

Useful websites

Flying Start England http://www.flyingstartengland.nhs.uk/preceptor-qualities.htm

FoNS Centre for Nursing Innovation http://www.fons.org/

Mind Tools http://www.mindtools.com/

National Leadership Council http://www.nhsleadership.org.uk/

NHS Employers Agenda for Change http://www.nhsemployers.org/PayAndContracts/AgendaForChange/Pages/Afc-Homepage.aspx

Nursing and Midwifery Council http://www.nmc-uk.org

The Queen's Nursing Institute http://www.qni.org.uk/

Appendix

Chapter 8: Completed care plan for case scenario 1

Problem and actual (A) or potential (P)	Goal/objective	Implementation (interventions planned)	Evaluation	Review date
Mrs Brown is at increased risk of falls (A)	To minimize the risk of falls for Mrs Brown and to ensure the environment is as safe as possible.	Complete with Mrs Brown a falls risk assessment and refer if appropriate with consent to the falls clinic/falls specialist nurse for further assessment.	Falls risk assessment completed and referred to clinic 24/6/11.	8/7/11
		To ensure Mrs Brown is provided with education, support and advice to promote safe mobilization. Provide practical information of how to minimize risk of falls around the home such as removal of rugs and a commode by the bed at night time.	Ongoing	30/6/11
			Manual handling risk assessment completed.	8/7/11
		Discuss and seek consent from Mrs Brown for a referral to both the OT and physiotherapist (this could be accessed via the falls clinic if referred) for assessments to educate, promote safety within the home and consider possible adaptations and aids to mobilize safely including footwear.	Will access allied health care professionals via falls clinic. Referral made for lifeline 24.6.11. Evie provided consent for key safe to home.	8/7/11
		Request a full medication review by Mrs Brown's GP. Last medication review was seven months ago.	Referral made to GP 23/6/11.	30/6/11

(Continued)

Chapter 8: Completed care plan for case scenario 1 (Continued)

Problem and actual (A) or potential (P)	Goal/objective	Implementation (interventions planned)	Evaluation	Review date
Mrs Brown is at risk of developing pressure ulcers (P)	Mrs Brown will not develop any pressure ulcers and skin integrity will be maintained.	Complete a pressure ulcer risk assessment and take appropriate action with consent of Mrs Brown.	Waterlow risk assessment completed. Pressure relieving mattress and chair cushion provided.	30/6/11
		Provide education and information relating to how to prevent and reduce the risk of Evie's skin 'breaking down', including change of position and care of Evie's skin.	Ongoing	30/6/11
		Provide nutritional education and ensure appropriate pressure relieving aids are provided.	Ongoing	30/6/11
		Advise Evie to change her position and promote mobilization at least every two hours, however this should be judged on an individual basis and may require a more frequent intervention if Evie's skin should discolour or show signs of non-blanching.		30/6/11
Mrs Brown has sustained a small skin tear on her left ankle	To promote Mrs Brown's wound to heal and minimize the risk of infection.	Complete a comprehensive wound assessment and appropriate documentation and involve Mrs Brown in the wound care planning process (including appropriate education).	Ongoing	30/6/11

Problem/Need	Goal	Action	Evaluation	Date
Mrs Brown recently has become forgetful and requires aids to effectively communicate (A)	Mrs Brown will be able to engage and actively participate in effective communication.	Dress and review Mrs Brown's wound according to her wound management chart. Report and record the progress of wound healing and any significant changes and take appropriate action.		
		When communicating Mrs Brown is aware that she requires to wear glasses and a hearing aid in her left ear.	Ongoing	8/7/11
		Attempt to sit in front of Mrs Brown when possible and speak clearly and at a slow pace.		
		Mrs Brown enjoys using her computer and emails so may benefit from accessing information and support from recommended Internet sites.	Referral made.	8/7/11
		Discuss with Mrs Brown and Elizabeth the opportunity to be referred to a memory specialist and consider the appropriateness of memory loss clinics.	Ongoing but using written prompts and verbal prompts by Elizabeth.	8/7/11
		Explore practical suggestions to support Evie and memory loss such as prompts from Elizabeth, written reminders in prominent places, watches/clocks with timers to prompt.	Blood test completed 24/6/11 and awaiting results.	30/6/11

(Continued)

Chapter 8: Completed care plan for case scenario 1 (*Continued*)

		For a full blood screen to be completed and GP to take appropriate action after discussion with Evie and Elizabeth. If appropriate refer to neurologist to investigate further memory loss and access support services such as the Admiral nurses (will support Elizabeth in her caring capacity). Also consider voluntary and independent organizations for respite breaks and social networking.	
Mrs Brown requires promoting to remind her to eat and drink (P)	Mrs Brown will maintain a satisfactory nutritional and fluid intake with a body mass index (BMI) within acceptable parameters.	Nutritional screening requires completion and appropriate action taken which may include a referral to a dietician or promotion of prescribed nutritional supplements if required.	Risk assessment completed and referral to community dietician made. 8/7/11
		Support and advice to be provided re a balanced nutritional and adequate fluid intake by the community nurses/dietician when required.	Ongoing 30/6/11
		Elizabeth prepares snacks for Evie throughout the day with a flask of tea and juice and telephones her if not there to promote Evie to take these. Elizabeth is able to ascertain what Evie likes to eat and promote choice. The suggestion of a delivery of hot meals has been made but offer declined at this present time. Elizabeth also supports Evie to clean her dentures and promotes mouth care. Evie cannot chew on her food without her dentures.	

Problem	Goal	Nursing action	Evaluation	Date
Mrs Brown is at risk of constipation (P)	Mrs Brown to maintain her normal elimination pattern.	Complete a bowel assessment with Mrs Brown and take appropriate action. Provide health education information in relation to fluid, nutritional intake and mobility. Elizabeth to support Evie to administer prescribed laxatives if her bowels are not open after three days. The commode will be nearby during the night for convenience and to reduce the risk of falls.	Assessment completed and continue with current routine.	15/7/11
Mrs Brown requires assistance of her paid carer to meet her personal hygiene needs (A)	Mrs Brown to state that her personal care needs have been met to an acceptable level.	Mrs Brown's formal carer visits every morning to assist Evie with washing and dressing, application of make up but promotes Evie's independence. Mrs Brown has her hair washed twice weekly with a mobile hairdresser visiting fortnightly. The chiropodist visits once a month to care for Evie's feet. The carer will observe for any changes in skin integrity, document and report any concerns to Elizabeth or the community nurses at the earliest opportunity. Both Evie's formal carer and her daughter Elizabeth will assist Evie to adjust bed linen/clothing according to maintain Evie's body temperature.	To continue	15/7/11

(Continued)

Chapter 8: Completed care plan for case scenario 1 (*Continued*)

Problem and actual (A) or potential (P)	Goal/objective	Implementation (interventions planned)	Evaluation	Review date
Mrs Brown feels low in mood that she is not able to participate as fully with social activities due to her forgetfulness and has missed her membership to the Castlefields residents group (A)	To acknowledge Mrs Brown's mental health issues and promote renewal of her social identity within the community and as an individual.	In partnership with Mrs Brown complete a depression screening assessment and with consent refer to GP and then for appropriate referral if required.	Depression screening completed and referred to GP.	8/7/11
		Encourage Mrs Brown to continue to engage via email with her friends and social networking. Possibly consider inviting members of the Castlefields residents group to her home or for her friend Bill to collect and take Mrs Brown to the meetings.	Ongoing support and Elizabeth invited residents for tea party at home address.	8/7/11
		Consider a social services referral to assess for assistance and accessibility to day services/voluntary and independent sector organizations.	Social services referral made 24/6/11 and to check progress.	30/6/11
Mrs Brown is concerned that the deterioration in her general health and mental well-being may be 'the beginning of the end' and 'would she die?' (A)	To discuss any issues and concerns Mrs Brown and Elizabeth may have at present in relation to dying and a diagnosis when obtained.	To identify the primary concerns that Mrs Brown and her daughter may have and address these or refer if appropriate.	To discuss further next visit.	30/6/11
		Reassure that any decision is always made in partnership and ultimately this remains the individual's choice.	Review with GP after blood test results back.	30/6/11
		Explain that when/if a diagnosis is obtained further discussions could be facilitated.	Integrate into discussion next visit.	30/6/11
		Take an appropriate opportunity and a sensitive approach to discuss and record and share Mrs Brown's wishes and preferences in relation to dying and engage with the advanced life planning process.		

Completed care plan for case scenario 2

Problem and actual (A) or potential (P)	Goal/objective	Implementation (interventions planned)	Evaluation	Review date
Essie is experiencing reduced mobility (A)	Essie to mobilize safely and the risk of falls to be kept to a minimum.	Complete a manual handling and falls risk assessment and take appropriate action.	Both completed and consent given for request of commode. To revaluate in a timely manner for Essie's bed to be raised and electric hoist/monkey pole to be requested. Refer to manual handling team for carer education with use of equipment.	8/7/11
		Discuss and seek consent from Essie for both an occupational therapist (OT) and physiotherapist (PT) referral for assessment. This is to include assessment of: Essie mobilizing with a stick and footwear; Essie's eligibility for a wheelchair; adaptations within the home;	Referral made to OT and PT 24/6/11.	30/6/11
		Essie managing the stairs within her house; Appropriateness for downstairs living/stair rail; Medication review.	Referral made to GP 24/6/11.	30/6/11
		Request disability blue badge application for car parking.	Referred to Macmillan nurse 24/6/11.	30.6.11

(Continued)

Completed care plan for case scenario 2 (Continued)

Problem and actual (A) or potential (P)	Goal/objective	Implementation (interventions planned)	Evaluation	Review date
Essie is at risk of developing pressure ulcers (P)	Essie will not develop any pressure ulcers and skin integrity will be maintained.	Promote safety when mobilizing and provide education in relation to possible neuropathy, changes in balance and immune suppression with increased infection risk.	Ongoing	30.6.11
		Complete a pressure ulcer risk assessment and take appropriate action with Essie's consent. Provide education and information to both Essie and Marvin relating to how to prevent and reduce the risk of Essie's skin 'breaking down', including change of position and care of Essie's skin especially with the chemotherapy where it may become dry and/or discoloured. Provide nutritional education and ensure appropriate pressure relieving aids are provided.	Waterlow risk assessment completed 23/6/11. Both a pressure relieving mattress and cushion have been requested and see above for manual handling equipment.	
		Advise Essie to change her position and promote mobilization at least every two hours, however this should be judged on an individual basis and may require a more frequent intervention if Essie's skin should discolour or show signs of non-blanching.		
Essie requires assistance to maintain her personal care needs (A)	Essie to state that her personal care needs have been met to an acceptable standard.	Marvin assists Essie with washing and dressing, care of hair and maintaining body temperature but Essie is independent washing some areas such as face, hands and intimate areas and cleaning her own teeth and applying her makeup.	Ongoing but awaiting social services assessment. Referral made 24.6.11.	8.7.11 8.7.11

Problem	Goal	Nursing action	Frequency	Date
		Both have consented to a referral to social services for assessment for care support and financial advice. Education provided to both Essie and Marvin in relation to observation for changes in skin integrity and possible mouth ulcers, nails or hair loss (in regards to possible side effects from chemotherapy) and to inform community nurses as soon as possible with any concerns.	Ongoing	30.6.11
Essie may develop difficulty with breathing as a side effect from her chemotherapy treatment and any deterioration in her condition (A)	Any side effects to be minimized to an acceptable level for Essie.	Education provided to Essie re the possible side effects such as tiredness, lethargy (currently experiencing), dizziness, aching muscles and joints, shortness of breath.	Ongoing	8.7.11
		To promote the use of breathing exercises to alleviate associated feelings of anxiety with these problems.	Monthly	24.7.11
		Review haemoglobin levels as directed by the oncology department and appropriate action to be taken to manage symptoms.	Information provided 24.6.11	24.7.11
		Provide support for Essie and information re voluntary/independent organizations to provide respite and assistance. Consider time management with Essie and how she may change her normal routine to accommodate changes in her health status.	Ongoing	30.6.11
Essie is at risk of constipation (P)	Essie to maintain her normal elimination pattern.	Complete a bowel assessment with Essie and take appropriate action. Essie is aware she may experience diarrhoea as a side effect of chemotherapy. Provide health education information in relation to fluid, nutritional intake and mobility.	Completed 24.6.11	8.7.11

(Continued)

Completed care plan for case scenario 2 (Continued)

Problem and actual (A) or potential (P)	Goal/objective	Implementation (interventions planned)	Evaluation	Review date
		Essie uses the downstairs toilet and a commode has been requested if required by Essie during the night for convenience and to reduce risk of falls.		
		Essie will self administer prescribed laxatives if her bowels are not open after three days.		
Essie is experiencing a decreased appetite (A)	Essie will maintain a satisfactory nutritional and fluid intake when possible.	Essie has been assessed by the community dietician previously and she has prescribed nutritional supplement drinks – three per day.	Community dietician visits Essie fortnightly for review.	28.6.11
		Community nurses to support community dietician and Essie and liaises with the nutritional support plan in place.	Ongoing	30.6.11
		Essie is aware that as her condition deteriorates her appetite may reduce further. Professionals will work to support Essie and review her care accordingly. This will include support with possible side effects of treatment such as altered taste, possible mouth ulcers and management of symptoms such as nausea and vomiting.		
Essie is experiencing difficulty adjusting to her altered body image after her left mastectomy (A)	For Essie to receive support through this transitional period.	The oncology team and breast care specialist nurses and community nurses are providing Essie and Marvin with continued support.	Ongoing – physically the wound has healed and no keloid scarring present. Psychologically support continues.	30.6.11

Problem/Need	Goal	Action/Intervention	Evaluation	Date
		Chemotherapy treatment is due to commence 4.7.11.	Review and collaboration with professionals and Essie ongoing.	5.7.11
Essie experiences interrupted sleep patterns (P)	For Essie to maintain a routine that is acceptable to her.	Essie and Marvin sleep separately to accommodate her altered sleep patterns. She does not take any medications but often reads. Support will continue to be provided as these patterns may be exacerbated or change as a side effect of her treatment.		5.7.11
Essie is aware that her prognosis is poor, treatment is palliative and that her condition will continue to deteriorate	To manage and alleviate Essie symptoms and anxieties to an acceptable level for her.	Discuss Essie's wishes and preferences in relation to future care planning and in partnership with Marvin.	Ongoing	30.6.11
		Essie has expressed a wish to die at home and community nurses will work with them and other professionals to facilitate this. Contact Macmillan nurses/palliative care team to initiate visit (Essie provided consent).	Referral made 24.6.11 and they will contact Essie to arrange visit.	Completed 24.6.11
		Refer Marvin for counselling as he has requested.	Referral made.	8.7.11
		Ensure Essie and Marvin are aware of who and how to contact appropriate professionals both in and out of hours service.	Details provided 23.6.11.	Completed 23.6.11
		Provide details of voluntary and independent organizations that may support Essie and Marvin with provision of respite services. Refer to continuing care for assessment for full NHS funding and fast tracking of application.	Individual needs portrayal to be completed with social services – date to be confirmed.	30.6.11

Chapter 10: Answer to Limestreet Immunisation Schedule

When to immunize	What is given	Vaccine and how it is given
2 months old	Diphtheria, tetanus, pertussis, polio and haemophilus influenzae type b (DTaP/IPV/Hib)	One injection (Pediacel)
	Pneumococcal (PCV)	One injection (Prevenar)
3 months old	Diphtheria, tetanus, pertussis, polio and haemophilus influenzae type b (DTaP/IPV/Hib)	One injection (Pediacel)
	Meningitis C (MenC)	One injection (Neisvac C or Meningitec or Menjugate)
4 months old	Diphtheria, tetanus, pertussis, polio and Haemophilus influenzae type b (DTaP/IPV/Hib)	One injection (Pediacel)
	Pneumococcal (PCV)	One injection (Prevenar)
Between 12 and 13 months old within a month of the first birthday	Haemophilus influenzae type b, Meningitis C (Hib/MenC)	One injection (Menitorix)
	Measles, mumps and rubella (MMR)	One injection (Priorix or MMRvaxPro)
	Pneumococcal (PCV)	One injection (Prevenar)
3 years 4 months to 5 years old	Diphtheria, tetanus, pertussis and polio (dTaP/IPV or DTaP/IPV)	One injection (Repevax or Infanrix-IPV)
	Measles, mumps and rubella (MMR)	One injection (Priorix or MMRvaxPro)

Index

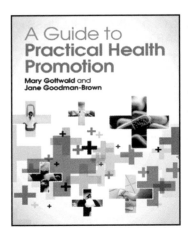

A GUIDE TO PRACTICAL HEALTH PROMOTION

Mary Gottwald and Jane Goodman-Brown

9780335244591 (Paperback)
August 2012

eBook also available

Do you have difficulties deciding which health promotion activities facilitate behavioural change?

This accessible book focuses on the practical activity of health promotion and shows students and practitioners how to actually apply health promotion in practice. The book uses case scenarios to explore how health promotion activities can empower individuals to make decisions that change their health related behaviour

Key features:

- Each chapter uses classic case studies in health promotion
- Includes lists, key points and other succinct tools to give the reader guidance
- Contains activities and specific tasks that can be used in practice

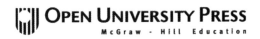

www.openup.co.uk

OPEN UNIVERSITY PRESS
McGraw - Hill Education

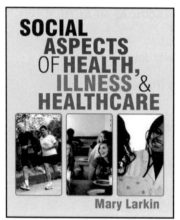

SOCIAL ASPECTS OF HEALTH, ILLNESS AND HEALTHCARE

Mary Larkin

9780335236626 (Paperback)
2011

eBook also available

This core textbook is the ideal companion text for health students studying social aspects of health and illness, whether it is part of a health studies degree or for a nursing or other professional qualification. Written at introductory level this is key reading for health students coming to the subject for the first time and looking for a broad and practical text.

Key features:

- Provides clear explanations of key concepts, extracts from primary sources, case studies and activities for study
- Explores and explains the different relationships between social categories and health
- Examines the role of the healthcare provider in society

www.openup.co.uk

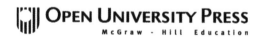

OPEN UNIVERSITY PRESS
McGraw - Hill Education

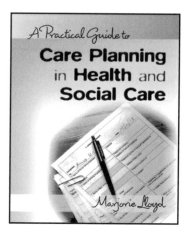

**A PRACTICAL GUIDE TO CARE PLANNING
IN HEALTH AND SOCIAL CARE**

Marjorie Lloyd

9780335237326 (Paperback)
2010

eBook also available

*"This is an excellent book for anyone starting out on the Common
Foundation year of their nursing degree, and as a reference to those further
into their degree, on placement, or newly qualified. The care planning
process is very well introduced using models and frameworks of care, with
thorough explanations and visual aids ... I would have no hesitation in
recommending this book to fellow students and colleagues, and I will use it
through the remainder of my degree and beyond."*
Conor Hamilton, Student Nurse, Queens University Belfast, UK

Key features:

- Interprofessional working
- Risk management
- Communication and listening skills

www.openup.co.uk

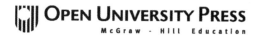

OPEN UNIVERSITY PRESS
McGraw - Hill Education

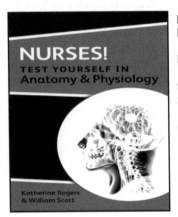

NURSES! TEST YOURSELF IN ANATOMY & PHYSIOLOGY

Katherine Rogers and William Scott

9780335241637 (Paperback)
2011

eBook also available

Looking for a quick and effective way to revise and test your knowledge? This handy book is the essential self-test resource for nurses studying basic anatomy & physiology and preparing for exams. This book includes over 450 questions in total, each with fully explained answers.

Key features:

- Organised into body systems chapters
- Includes a range of question types
- Provides a list of clearly explained answers to questions

www.openup.co.uk

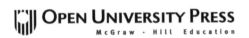

OPEN UNIVERSITY PRESS
McGraw · Hill Education

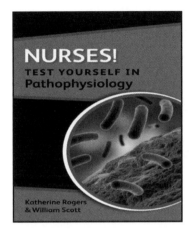

NURSES! TEST YOURSELF IN PATHOPHYSIOLOGY

Katherine Rogers and William Scott

9780335242238 (Paperback)
2011

eBook also available

Looking for a quick and effective way to revise and test your knowledge?
This handy book is the essential self-test resource to help nurses revise and
prepare for their pathophysiology exams. The book covers a broad range of
conditions common to nursing practice including pneumonia, diabetes, asthma,
eczema and more. The book includes over 300 questions and 70 glossary terms
in total.

Key features:

- Organised into body systems chapters
- Includes a range of question types
- Provides a list of clearly explained answers to questions

www.openup.co.uk

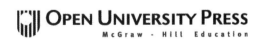

OPEN UNIVERSITY PRESS
McGraw - Hill Education

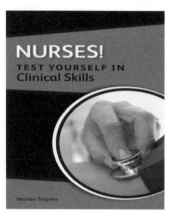

NURSES! TEST YOURSELF IN CLINICAL SKILLS

Marian Traynor

9780335244836 (Paperback)
October 2012

eBook also available

This book provides nursing students with a sound knowledge of clinical skills that will prepare them for the reality of clinical practice in order to be safe and effective practitioners at the point of registration.
The book is organised into chapters that address different groups of skills, and includes chapters on: Infection control, Respiratory Skills, Cardiovascular Skills, Neuro assessment skills, Early Warning Scores (observations) and Drug Admin.

Key features:

- Includes a range of question types plus a labelling exercise that reflects those used in real exams
- Answers are explained clearly so students can see where they went right or wrong
- Can be used both for self-testing and more constructive revision

www.openup.co.uk

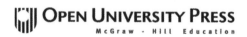